PRAISE FOR *THE WAY OF THE HAPPY WOMAN*

"With insight and accessibility, Sara Avant Stover invites us to pull together the essential ingredients for living an intentional life, one we might truly call happy. *The Way of the Happy Woman* invites, encourages, supports, and celebrates women coming home to themselves in the body, heart, and mind. If a book can act as a spiritual friend, this one does."

— Sarah Powers, author of *Insight Yoga*

"*The Way of the Happy Woman* knocked my socks off! As a woman who already considers herself pretty 'healthy' and 'connected,' I was blown wide open with how vast and fruitful the possibilities for living a full and feminine life really are. Sara Avant Stover's intimate writing style, tremendous wit and compassion, and in-depth knowledge of women's bodies and emotional health have yielded a phenomenally life-altering piece of work. I will buy this book for my mother, my sister, my daughter, and all my girlfriends this year!"

— Peach Friedman, author of *Diary of an Exercise Addict*

"From the first page of *The Way of the Happy Woman*, I breathed a great sigh of relief. As women we are told to be warriors, smart, sexy, successful. We can have it all, but at what price? It seems all we really want is to be happy. Thank you, Sara, for helping us remember our true divine nature and making it so accessible."

— Nischala Joy Devi, author of *The Secret Power of Yoga*
and *The Healing Path of Yoga*

"In a time when women are running themselves ragged juggling their career, family, and more, Sara's soothing words of wisdom remind us to slow down and pay attention to what really matters — health and happiness. *The Way of the Happy Woman*'s simple and practical suggestions will help you nourish your mind, body, and soul with mindfulness and compassion every day of the year."

— Jennifer Lee, author of *The Right-Brain Business Plan*

"In poetic prose with the tender touch of a wise older sister, Sara Avant Stover offers up tips and tricks for simple, beauty-filled, mindful living. This book will cause you to rest, reflect, and rejoice all at once!"

— Kimberly Wilson, author of *Hip Tranquil Chick* and *Tranquilista*

"Sara Avant Stover walks her talk. She knows suffering and has found a down-to-earth, practical, and uplifting way through it, which she offers here. This wonderful book is a must-read for every woman in search of greater happiness. Sara shows us that happiness is absolutely possible!"
— Ed and Deb Shapiro, award-winning authors of *Be the Change*

"It is pure pleasure to dive into this well-written and inspiring book full of tips, recipes, and practices for radiant and happy living. It feels like I have in my hands a box of chocolate for the soul."
— Chameli Ardagh, founder of AwakeningWomen.com

"With inspiring vision, Sara Avant Stover offers supportive, practical, and fun body-mind solutions to help women stay healthy throughout the year."
— Bobby Clennell, author and illustrator of *The Woman's Yoga Book* and *Watch Me Do Yoga*

THE WAY
of the
HAPPY
WOMAN

Living the Best Year
of Your Life

SARA AVANT STOVER

FOREWORD BY JENNIFER LOUDEN
PREFACE BY KATE NORTHRUP MOLLER

New World Library
Novato, California

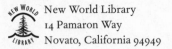

New World Library
14 Pamaron Way
Novato, California 94949

Illustrations by Molly O'Brien
Text design by Tona Pearce Myers
Library of Congress Cataloging-in-Publication Data
Stover, Sara Avant, date.
 The way of the happy woman : living the best year of your life / Sara Avant Stover ; foreword by Jennifer Louden ; preface by Kate Northrup Moller.
    p.   cm.
 Includes bibliographical references.
 ISBN 978-1-57731-982-5 (pbk.)
 1. Women—Health and hygiene. 2. Self-care, Health. I. Title.
 RA778.S829 2011
 613'.04244—dc22   2011006706

First printing, May 2011
ISBN 978-1-57731-982-5
Printed in the United States on 100% postconsumer-waste recycled paper

New World Library is a proud member of the Green Press Initiative.

10 9 8 7 6 5 4 3

For my grandmother, Sara Avant Hatton.
Thank you for seeing me and for always telling me what a beautiful writer I am.

For the healing, empowerment, and delight
of the seven generations of women both before and after me.

And for the Divine Mother, who wrote this book through me.

WHEN I AM AMONG THE TREES

When I am among the trees,
especially the willows and the honey locust,
equally the beech, the oaks and the pines,
they give off such hints of gladness.
I would almost say that they save me, and daily.

I am so distant from the hope of myself,
in which I have goodness, and discernment,
and never hurry through the world
    but walk slowly, and bow often.

Around me the trees stir in their leaves
and call out, "Stay awhile."
The light flows from their branches.

And they call again, "It's simple," they say,
"and you too have come
into the world to do this, to go easy, to be filled
with light, and to shine."

— MARY OLIVER

Another world is not only possible, she's on her way...
on a quiet day, if I listen very carefully, I can hear her breathing.
— ARUNDHATI ROY

If we forget, we can remember again.
— DR. CLARISSA PINKOLA ESTÉS

Women play a pivotal role in the enlightenment and upliftment
of a moral society. Their power grows from their investment in preserving
the sacred ways of nature. It is this power that makes women the great
educators, guides, instructors, and nourishers for their men and children.
At this axial time in the history of the earth, it is imperative that women
reclaim and resume their roles as nurturers, healers, and the healed.
— MAYA TIWARI

Contents

PART 5: WINTER

Foreword

As I read the first few pages of this book, I sighed with relief. Thank goodness it isn't about taking on some big ding-dang-do self-improvement plan or eating only raw food while standing on my head or otherwise improving myself. I learned a long time ago that the only problem with self-improvement is...it doesn't work.

What *does* work is honoring ourselves, trusting ourselves, celebrating ourselves, meeting ourselves where we are, how we are. I did it this morning: I was angry at myself for eating sugar for days (I typically get depressed if I even look at sugar) because I was sad about my daughter's leaving for college (in a year and a half, but yeah, she's my only), so I started to make elaborate plans to never eat sugar again and get up at 5 A.M. and chant the Gayatri Mantra 108 times and...and then I wrapped my arms around myself, gave myself a big hug, and loved myself as my itchy, depressed, gassy, neurotic self. In that simple gesture, my sanity and freedom were restored, and I could choose my actions from there.

This book is about wrapping your arms around yourself in a thousand different delicious, embodied ways. This is sacred self-care, and doing it is urgently important. You've probably noticed that the world isn't doing so well. Climate change is affecting all of us now (experienced a big storm or a weird heat wave lately?), and these changes demand that we change how we live. The situation is dire, yes, and by facing the direness, we can find the energy for change.

Only we can't change anything if we are paralyzed by fear, frozen in self-hatred, comatose and sick from eating fake food, or living three feet above our heads, pretending we don't have a body. Self-care opens the pathways for the energy, insight, and determination we need to face up to our global plight and find our particular way to make a difference.

Plus, there's a bonus to sacred self-care, and who doesn't love a bonus (remember the prize in the cereal box?) — when you hold something precious, you naturally want to protect it. It's your animal nature to do this. If you come to love yourself so richly and deeply (and maybe you already do — hallelujah), you are then invited to connect that self-love to world-love in very practical ways that are also life-giving and fun. Stand back, darling, you really will save the world.

Don't get me wrong — I'm not saying that all you need to do is follow some of Sara Avant Stover's enticing ideas, and you've done your bit. On that note, I love the story that Nobel Peace Prize–winner and land-mine activist Jody Williams tells in her TED talk. She was sitting on a dais in front of thousands of people with eight other Nobel laureates, including the Dalai Lama, waiting her turn to speak, when the Dalai Lama leaned over and whispered, "Jody, I'm a Buddhist monk." "Yes, your Holiness," Jody said, "Your robe gives it away." (You can just imagine him giggling, can't you?) "You know I like meditation and I pray. But I have become skeptical. I do not believe meditation and prayer will change this world. I think what we need is action."

As always, the Dalai Lama cuts right to the truth: action is needed, and needed now, from every single one of us. The action you take is nourished and inspired by meditation and prayer and Downward-Facing Dog and green smoothies and beautiful books like this one. These tools may also help you discern what action is yours to take, and — perhaps most of all — they will give you skin in the game. Because when you practice the lifestyle Sara offers here, you connect daily with your longing to make the world an equitable and sustainable place. You connect through your arms, legs, mouth, breath, and mind with your desire for all beings to have peace, safety, happiness, and green smoothies. And because you are connecting by practicing sacred self-care, your desire to serve will not burn you out or overwhelm you but will become part of your self-care, inspiring you to take even better care of yourself so you can better serve.

I live every single day with a fierce longing in me, a longing that pushes me, prods me, tantalizes me — a desire that flames at the back of my heart, an itch I can never quite scratch. It's a longing to help make a better world, to fully live this one precious life I have, to be sure everyone gets a chance to live fully. Honestly, I don't always really know what this longing is, only that it is, and I believe you feel it too.

I used to use books like this one to try to make the longing go away — to fix it or to finally *understand* it. I understand now that the longing I feel is never going away. *It's not supposed to.* It's a divine itch, and our job is to use it to be of service in a way that gives voice to it: to use it as fuel to keep going. To use it to find the courage to bring our genius to the world.

These days, I take in the ancient wisdom and expansive love that Sara and other teachers offer, to create a setting for the jewel of my longing. A way to frame it, steady it, support it, and connect to it. I use self-care and spiritual practice to help me bear the longing I feel so it can work on me and through me. That's very different from trying to fix something or make myself better.

If all of this sounds a bit much, here's the simple truth: do more of what Sara offers you in this book, in a spirit of openness and self-acceptance, and you will have more energy and bandwidth to take action on behalf of what you most care about — whatever that may be. Share these ideas with your friends and children and sweethearts, and that energy and bandwidth will spread too. Do it all in the spirit of gentle curiosity, with the knowledge that you can always begin again. And please, above all, have fun.

I toast you with a green smoothie while we change the world!

Jennifer Louden, author of
The Life Organizer and *The Woman's Comfort Book*

Sara Avant Stover's request for me to write the preface to this beautiful book arrived on the day I left for the indefinite road trip that I'm affectionately calling the Freedom Tour. Within a week I had sold or given away the vast majority of my possessions, left New York City in a U-Haul in a snowstorm, and flown to Ellicottville, New York, to pick up my new home, a little white Toyota Prius. In the craziness of that transition, Sara's email slipped through the cracks. It wasn't until two weeks, thirteen states, and 4,200 miles later that I saw Sara's email in the bottom of my constantly overflowing in-box. I was simultaneously honored by the request and mortified that it had taken me two weeks to respond.

Without giving it much thought, as is generally the case when I have an immediate gut feeling about something, I responded to Sara's request with an enthusiastic "Yes!" I pressed send as I rolled into Boulder, Colorado, on day sixteen of the Freedom Tour. Forty-two minutes later I received her reply that she lived in Boulder and perhaps we could meet for tea in two days. The universe works in mysterious ways. I knew immediately that the connection between us had a bit of extra sparkle and shine.

As soon as I opened Sara's manuscript and began reading her story, I was struck by the synchronicity of the two of us connecting. Her story mirrors twists and turns that I've been through in my own life. As with many universal truths, it was deliciously uncanny to read. As a fellow Ivy League–educated dancer, I found Sara's story of getting a wake-up call that forced her to get back in touch with her inner wisdom more than familiar. Her willingness to listen to the truth her body was telling her and make a dramatic change to save her own life speaks to me deeply, and I know it will touch countless other women as well.

Sara left New York City in her twenties to live in Thailand and discover a lush, fertile, wise way of living that her feminine wisdom already knew the recipe for. That recipe had simply been misplaced in the milieu of high-achievement, perfectionist living. Similarly, urged by the callings of my intuition, at the age of twenty-seven I just got rid of everything and left New York City on an indefinite journey whose final destination is yet to be seen.

Sara and I stand on the shoulders of the generations of women who came before us. Our path to listening to our bodies' wisdom, taking the time to discover who we truly are, and allowing ourselves to tell the truth has been paved by the struggles and victories of our mothers, grandmothers, and great-grandmothers. The moment I read the dedication to this book acknowledging the seven generations before and after us, I knew that Sara and I were on the same page. The reason that we have the luxury of spending time in self-discovery mode — whether in Thailand, on a road trip, or in our own hometowns — is because our foremothers (such as my biological mother, Dr. Christiane Northrup, and others such as Gloria Steinem, Clarissa Pinkola Estés, and Gail Straub) have unlocked the doors for us.

I think I speak for not only Sara and myself but also our entire generation when I say that we feel deep gratitude for those who have come before us. I grew up the daughter of a woman known for the waves and triumphs she'd made in the field of women's health, particularly for midlife women. I've spent time around and heard the stories of many, many women of the baby boomer generation — women in my mother's practice, women I've met in workshops, and hundreds of others I've worked with in Team Northrup. Their stories are about transformation, about the process of remembering the truth of themselves through the wisdom of their bodies. Many of these women had to endure sexism, financial upheaval, emotional or physical abuse, miserable marriages, difficult pregnancies, and feelings of loneliness and self-loss while raising families and navigating the often competing roles of women as mothers, daughters, lovers, wives, friends, business owners, seekers, leaders, activists, and human beings. Many of these women didn't discover the ability, wherewithal, and freedom to heed the wake-up calls of their bodies until midlife.

The women of Sara's and my generation have the luxury of heeding these wake-up calls earlier. The women who have come before us have given us the permission to not wait until midlife to begin to listen to our bodies. This book could not exist if it weren't for women such as my mother and her peers. Sara was able to transform and live her life from the inside out rather than the outside in — without having to wait until halfway through her life — because of the pre-tread paths upon which she is able to walk. I was able to get rid of my home and my possessions and let go of my life as I knew it because of the solid foundation I'm blessed enough to stand on.

So I thank the generations of women who have come before, I thank Sara for walking a parallel path with me as a woman "waking up early," and I plant the seed for the generations of women who will come after us to be able to heed their wake-up calls earlier and earlier. Here's to having more time on the planet living the truth of who we really are. Here's to putting our rudder in the water and steering our course from the messages we receive from within. Here's to these experiences becoming the new norm rather than the exception to the rule.

It's no coincidence that you have found yourself with this book in your hands, just as it was no coincidence that Sara asked me to write this preface for her or that, unbeknownst to me, I responded to her request two weeks late but at the perfect time, as I was driving into the very city where she lives. It's no coincidence that Sara and I come from similar backgrounds and each felt we needed to leave New York City to seek the answers we ultimately knew were within us, and that we needed to simplify, slow down, and reduce the static in order to hear them.

Your body knows the answers already. She has led you to pick up this book. She is the only one you get this lifetime. You are the only one going all the way with you this time around. Follow Sara's refreshing guidance to incorporate only what resonates with you in this book instead of attacking it like a new program, some sort of regimen to whip yourself into shape, or adding it to your already full to-do list. Your body thrives on love. Treat her as the divine creature she is, and I promise, she will never steer you wrong.

Let Sara's courage be your guiding light. Let her willingness to go to the dark spots and dip into the shadowy places be your assurance that it's safe to go there as well. "The darkest nights yield the most luminous dawns," she writes. Know that this journey with our female bodies is not about perfection or seeking only moments of joy and bliss. Seek your own contrast as Sara and the generations of women who have come before have already done. Live into what it means to create your life from your inner knowing, in three dramatic, full-relief dimensions, warts and all.

Sara is refreshingly honest and delightfully permissive in her urgings to not use this book to add to your busyness. She reminds us that we're whole right now. This journey as women is not about overhauling our lives or getting on a new program. Perhaps instead it's about stripping away layers rather than adding on. Hopefully, eventually, we will begin diving deeper into the truth of our divinity that pulsates just below the surface.

This book is a love letter to the feminine and a road map for you to find your way back to your home in your female body. It's not about giving you answers that you don't already have somewhere inside you or curing what ails you. Instead, it's about reminding you of what already lies inside. Sara guides us to true embodiment through being conscious about what we put into our bodies and how we move our bodies. It's so elegant and simple. She tells us, as I've always known but need constant reminders of, that a happy life comes from easing into our inner nature as well as taking cues from the natural world around us.

Sip the wisdom within these pages slowly. Swirl it around before you swallow. Notice what stirs inside you as you read Sara's words. Pay attention to the parts that make you cry, the parts that make you uncomfortable, and the parts that remind you of what you already know. As Sara takes you by the hand, enjoy this journey home.

— Kate Northrup Moller,
cocreator of Team Northrup (www.TeamNorthrup.com)

Introduction

He left the news on my answering machine. Like thieves, his words invaded me — stealing my ability to hide from the truth any longer. Twenty-one years old, I stood barefoot in my mother's Connecticut kitchen. The late-afternoon sunlight fell through the windows and onto the long, braided patterns of the wood floor beneath me. I felt both frozen and aged, all within a few moments, which normally would have whizzed by with the washing of dishes or the unpacking of groceries. I stood there, and a voice that seemed to know what this was all about rose up from inside me: "Whatever happens now, life will never be the same."

"Your pap smear results came back. They show abnormal cell growth on your cervix. I'm concerned. You'll have to come back in for a biopsy as soon as possible. Please call me back, and we'll set something up," my doctor announced.

It was April 1999, one month before my much-anticipated graduation from New York City's Barnard College. I had gone to the gynecologist as part of a litany of physical exams I needed to confirm my acceptance to serve as a health education volunteer with the Peace Corps in West Africa. Everything else had been approved, except this final test.

Later that week I did as my doctor advised. I went in for a biopsy and learned that I had cervical dysplasia, or the advanced precursor to cervical cancer — stage III, to be exact. I couldn't believe it. It was as if I were suddenly plummeting from the top of my own private universe. I had just been told I'd be graduating Phi Beta Kappa and summa cum laude. I practiced yoga, ran, and was a vegan. I looked healthy, perfect, really — on the outside. How could this be happening? To me?

Yet, inside, a secret part of me knew. Knew the sadness, the loneliness, the confusion, the torment I felt inside. Sometimes these feelings exploded to the surface when I was alone with my belly full, finger down my throat, heaving

I

over the toilet, hoping that no one would hear. I was the only one who bore the demands of my inner tyrant: "Do more," "Do it better," "You're not good enough." A smaller voice had whispered to me that this couldn't go on forever, that one day I'd have to face myself. Now its quiet urgings rang loud and clear. This was my wake-up call.

Shortly after the biopsy I returned to the doctor for a cryptoscopy, an attempt to freeze the irregular cells and stunt their growth. After the procedure, as I lay on the examining table with my legs spread, my doctor, at my feet, told me that I couldn't go to Africa. The healthcare there simply wasn't reliable enough. I would need to get a pap smear every three months to monitor my condition.

Going to Africa was my plan A *and* my plan B. "Please, please, is there anything I can do to help myself heal before then? What can I do?" I pleaded.

Without hesitation, he firmly answered, "The only thing you can do is wait and come back in three months. The details are up to you."

I felt deflated, stripped of my power and hope. My mother, who had come with me, ushered me out of the office and into the parking garage. Finally, my sobs broke through as she held me in her arms. I felt completely broken. "Sara, Sara, remember," she soothed, "when one door closes another one opens."

And, as is usually the case with mothers, she was right.

A few weeks later, out of the blue, over coffee at an Upper West Side pastry shop, a former high school dean offered me a job teaching English literature, writing, and dance at an international school in Chiang Mai, Thailand, where he would be serving as the headmaster. He told me I had forty-eight hours to get back to him with my reply.

Later that afternoon I rushed to a nearby bookstore and browsed through their Thailand travel guides. I knew nothing about Asia, but I quickly learned that the healthcare in Thailand was good and affordable, which meant I could get my required checkups. In my gut, it felt right.

FROM BREAKDOWN TO BREAKTHROUGH

I ended up living in northern Thailand for the next several years. The journey that ensued — in both my inner and outer worlds — is what led me to write this book. I entered a land filled with the tools I needed to heal and the sense of safety I needed to truly face myself. In later years, once I became a yoga teacher, Thailand, and my travels throughout the world, gifted me with opportunities to meet many other women, of all different ages and nationalities, who were suffering in similar ways.

After I arrived in Chiang Mai, it didn't take long for my type A, over-achieving New York City pace to slow down to match the hypnotic lull of Thailand's cicadas, afternoon thunderstorms, and banana leaves blowing in the breeze. The tempo suited me and reminded me that nature and I were one and the same. We lived in intimate rhythm with each other — a knowing I had lost long ago. Everyone napped after lunch. They smiled at me when I passed by on the street. While on a superficial level I thought I had been leading a healthy life before, my new surroundings showed me just how much I had been in denial, constantly trying to run from my inner pain. I did this by filling my days with so many "to-dos" and by being so obsessed with perfection that most of the time I was literally forgetting to breathe.

In Asia I traded my six-mile daily runs for long walks in the countryside. I sipped out of coconuts instead of Starbucks cups, and I opened to the abundance of healing wisdom around me: yoga, Traditional Chinese Medicine, Reiki, Ayurveda (the traditional medical system of India), chi gung, Buddhist insight meditation, traditional Thai massage, and detoxification programs that finally taught me how to trust and listen to my body. After a few months, my pap smears showed significant improvement, and, one year later, I had fully recovered.

In the ten years since, I have not only healed my precancerous cervix but also addressed my irregular menstruation, anorexia, bulimia, exercise addiction, insomnia, anxiety, and ovarian cysts — all of which I now know were contributors to my health scare. But the true cause was my disconnection from my body, my femininity, and nature herself. My life had been plagued by the constant, underlying discomfort of being alive as a woman, in a woman's body. I had felt melancholy, estranged from myself and others, and undeserving of true happiness. What I have discovered through my healing process, which continues to this day, is just how simple it is to be healthy, happy, and whole as a woman — and just how hard it can be to return to this essential truth amid the many mixed messages and complexities of our modern world.

I've met enough women to know that you too have a story. Maybe it's not as extreme as mine, or maybe it is more so, but at some level, you're ready to be healed, to thrive rather than to just survive, and to play your unique role in restoring the sacred balance on this planet through becoming more of who you are with love, grace, fierceness, and dignity. You too are hungry for a deeper connection with yourself and with those who fill your life; and you too want to remember what's truly important. You long to return to a simpler way of living, one that reminds you to slow down, simplify, value patient practice over quick fixes, care for yourself first, embrace your vulnerability as your greatest strength, and find true, lasting happiness within.

I would never trade my hardships — past, present, or future — for purely blissful encounters. These very tribulations have revealed what true happiness is. The darkest nights yield the most luminous dawns. If everything always went your way, you would be denied the precious opportunities to grow, surrender, trust, and evolve. Without fear you would never learn to be courageous. Without anger you would never learn forgiveness. Without heartbreak you would never open your heart to true love.

The red tents and moon lodges of our ancestors offered spaces in which to commune with other women while enduring these dark nights. Today we bear our pain alone, and we hardly even notice when the moon dissolves into darkness each month. We haven't learned how to harness the power of our emotions and intuition to steer us — and our communities — through life. Much of our collective emotional and physical suffering as women comes from the fast pace of modern living and centuries of denying the power of feminine wisdom. These factors complicate (and at times even eradicate) our connection to nature and her cycles. When living in or visiting a big city, one can go days, weeks, or even months without touching her bare feet to the ground or resting beneath the shady canopy of a tree. When I lived in New York City I rarely saw stars, and I never knew what phase the moon was in. We accept this as normal, but it's not. This doesn't mean that we need to abandon city living; it means we need to approach it in a radically new way. Modern times demand that we learn how to interweave ancient healing traditions into our urban realities. If we don't simplify, slow down, and start *feeling* our way through life more than *thinking* our way through it, we're going to get sick, tired, and angry — if we're not already.

YOU ARE THE ONE YOU'VE BEEN WAITING FOR

No doctor, spouse, TV personality, yoga instructor, or medicine woman can heal you. She can help support and inspire you, no doubt. She can show you the way. But ultimately you have to take the power back into your own hands and treat each moment as an opportunity to reclaim your health, and, in turn, your wholeness and happiness. Being healthy isn't about doing everything right and having everything go your way; rather, it is a way of being and perceiving yourself and the world with honesty — of showing up for life fully.

My healing crisis was a call from my spirit to wake up to the ways I was abusing myself, ignoring my soul, and disrupting the sacred balance of life, which as women we're here to maintain. It was a wake-up call to lead the life I was born to live, that deep down I ached to live.

When I finally listened, I could allow my passions and unique gifts — which have culminated in the writing of this book — to come forth. In the following pages I outline step-by-step the key lifestyle and embodiment practices I used to reclaim my innate happiness, health, and wholeness and to truly come home to myself as a woman. I have also shared these practices with women around the world for the past decade. I hope that they will be as beneficial to you as they have been to me and many others.

By coming along with me on this journey and participating in each season of the year, you will discover a whole new approach to living. You can embody this new way of being for the rest of your life and share it with those around you both directly and indirectly — through doing what you do and being who you are. The path that I lay out here ushers you directly into a more feminine approach to living, one that's guided from the inside out, bringing forth qualities such as compassion, beauty, sensuality, nurturance, creativity, and receptivity — all of which the world is in dire need of right now. The path restores your queenly dignity and indigenous earthly power. It reminds you of who you truly are.

You will learn how to lead a fulfilling life that's aligned with the cycles of the universe and that is guided from your heart. It's time to stop letting the demands of others dominate your life and to start trusting your own magnificence. It's time to stop ignoring nature and start trusting her and seeing what potent medicine she offers for your growth and healing every moment of every day.

These perks, as brilliant as they may be, are only secondary to the greatest gift that my journey has given me — the gift of self-love. Without it, true health and happiness aren't possible. That's why every page of this book guides you to embracing the self-love that you so deserve and that is there waiting inside you.

Love is the essence of who we are. At the end of our lives what really matters is the answer to the question, "How well did I love?" We feel love's powerful force in a flower growing through a sidewalk crack and a baby bursting forth from the birth canal. Life and beauty want to reign, against all odds. When we tap into the force of love, suddenly the unforgivable can be forgiven, the unhealable can be healed. The capacity for greatness in the human body, spirit, and heart is so much stronger than we give it credit for. As the famous line in the Talmud reminds us, "Every blade of grass has its angel that bends over it and whispers, 'Grow. Grow.' " We're always immersed in this beneficent, nurturing love. The question is, Do you recognize it? Do you listen? Do you allow yourself to receive it?

HOW THIS BOOK IS ORGANIZED

Through adapting the ancient tools of yoga, meditation, cooking, and balanced living for the modern woman's lifestyle, *The Way of the Happy Woman* returns us to simplicity, slowing down, aligning with nature's cycles, and living from the inside out to discover our indestructible inner happiness. Arranged in five parts, it explains how to reverse our disconnection from nature so that we know both the repercussions that come from living out of sync with the larger whole and, more important, what to do about it. Communing with our cycles is the foundation of a woman's health. Our hormonal cycles ebb and flow like the tides and the waxing and waning of the moon. Our emotions, creative urges, and life stages mirror nature's seasonal wheel from birth, to death, to rebirth. Healing ourselves requires healing our relationship to these biorhythms. That's why I structured this book according to the seasons of the year.

Part 1, "The Basics," outlines the core principles behind the Way that we'll be following throughout the year. The chapters in this section serve as the base camp for our journey, describing foundational practices that you can use during any season of the year. You'll also learn what supplies you need to stock up on for our journey together, how to set up a sacred space, and how to plan an ideal daily routine. In part 2, we begin in spring, the time of year for giving birth to fresh ways of being. In these chapters you'll discover what wants to come to life inside you and how to take steps to realize those dreams. Decluttering your living space, cleaning up and greening your diet, doing a one-day detox, and building your life force through dynamic movement are all practices that will help you to lighten up after a long winter and let your creative spirit soar. From spring we move into part 3, "Summer," which is about celebration and the blossoming into maturity. The vibrant flowers of this season burst forth from the soil of the springtime, which you fertilized with your clear creative intentions. It's in the summer when our dreams become realities and we can joyfully partake in them. As Elizabeth Gilbert wrote in *Eat, Pray, Love*, "You have to participate relentlessly in the manifestation of your own blessings."[1]

Through trying out the cooling summer recipes made of summer's abundant produce, connecting with our sexual, sensual self, bringing a spirit of play and vacation into each day, and learning new yoga practices to both quiet and excite us, we learn how to fully appreciate the abundance and expansiveness of this fleeting season.

The winds of autumn arrive in part 4, and here you learn the essential life lesson of letting go — both of summer's beauty and of relationships, projects, and parts of yourself that you've outgrown. The warming, robust recipes of the fall celebrate the harvest around you while fortifying your immune system for the winter season. Through yoga and meditation you'll learn to quell anxieties that arise from change and surrender and to deepen your self-confidence.

In part 5 we explore winter, a season whose significance we tend to overlook. You can't have a vibrant spring without the dormancy of winter, and in these chapters you'll learn how to slow down amid all the holiday hustle and bustle to incubate your heart's deepest dreams and desires — without falling into lethargy or depression. Nurturing winter foods energize you without adding excess weight, while the yoga and meditation practices keep your body and heart vibrantly tranquil and inspired to receive creative visions.

Before we start, I would like to say a few more essential things. First, the Way is not about perfection. It's not another way for you to fix yourself or to "get everything right." It's not another way for you to feel bad about yourself. Rather, it's about embracing and loving through all the kinks and idiosyncrasies that make you the irresistible and utterly lovable woman that you are. It's about being present and paying attention to the sacredness of the way the sun rises and sets each day and to everything that transpires in between those moments. You are already completely whole and healthy — that is your essence, the right and blessing you were born into. These practices serve only as reminders in case you've forgotten or lost touch with them. They're ancient rituals applied to modern times to help you reconnect with the shining jewel that you already are. As women we don't need one more excuse to berate ourselves! So use this book as a guide. A good girlfriend. An inspiration. Please feel my loving support and my deep care for you as we journey through this year together. That brings me to my second point, which is that this is not a system or a methodology. It's a personal process, so please apply only what works for you. Try it all out. Then discern what's relevant and what's not. Let your own experience be your teacher. Please don't get stressed out by this! We all have so much on our to-do lists already. The Chinese character for *busyness* translates as "heart killing." My intention in this book is to make your heart soar by helping you to slow down, simplify, and rest more at ease with yourself and your life. At times you may need to take a step back, breathe deeply, and revisit the big picture of what you really want from all of this.

Everything I share here I have learned from my own teachers and applied to my own life. If I have made mistakes or misrepresented these teachings, this reflects no fault of theirs but rather my own misunderstanding.

Whatever happens this year (and beyond), I'm certain that the outcomes will be far better, more magical, and more powerful than you and I alone could have ever imagined. As one of my favorite Chinese proverbs declares, "When women come together, they move mountains." So now I extend my hand to you in warm invitation. Are you ready? Let's move those mountains.

PART I

THE BASICS

Chapter 1

KEEP IT SIMPLE

I warn you — if you're looking for complicated, you've come to the wrong place. *The Way of the Happy Woman* heralds a return to the basics. There's an elegance to simplicity. It brings you to the heart of what really matters. Yet it contains a paradox as well. Being simple can be really difficult — at first. It hurts to change, to let go, and to trade in old, debilitating habits for new, more empowering ones. On the other hand, simplicity can be really easy. It calls you to strip away nonessentials to reveal who you truly are. There's something tremendously light and liberating about living from that place. So while you might feel you need to take many steps to lead the life of your dreams, a core part of you is already there.

You *are* health. You *are* happiness. These are your natural states. You already have the answers. You already have inside you everything you've ever wanted or looked for elsewhere. That's why you will find no elaborate rituals or convoluted dogma here. No shoulds or musts. No finish lines or prizes. Your unique process — and what you discover about yourself along the way — is the true reward. This process can get complex, however, since the essence of who you are often gets trampled on and covered over by your doubts, worries, and fears. It also gets denied every time you turn away from your inner wisdom, move too quickly through life, ignore your body, and cut yourself off from nature's rhythms.

LIVING FROM THE INSIDE OUT

Rushing around, adhering to overflowing schedules, and listening to demands dictated by some outside authority, we ignore our inner wisdom, our innate rhythms, and our intimate connection to nature's cycles. Instead of being slaves to others' demands, we need to start trusting and living from our own inner impulses. Otherwise, we'll never know how it feels to reside comfortably and confidently in our own skin, sovereign over ourselves.

Envision a woman in your life — past or present — who is at home in herself. How do you feel when she walks into the room? When she sits down next to you? When she speaks to you? Most likely she is not strikingly beautiful in the conventional sense, but her ease of being and the respect that she commands — simply by being authentically herself — make her glow with grace, elegance, and mystery. You too can feel at home. You too can be that woman.

Slowing down, listening, and doing less return us to our basic goodness, and only from there can we emerge stronger, brighter, and, well, happier. To truly survive and flourish as modern women, we need to start living from the inside out. For each time we fail to do so, we lead unfulfilled lives. And our hearts wither. Sometimes a little. Sometimes a lot.

> ## TRY THIS
>
> Make a list of all the things causing you stress right now. Include everything you can think of, big and small. Then, next to each item, write down how that particular stressful situation affects you. For example, if the stressor is "too many emails to answer," then next to it write, "anxiety, shortness of breath, pressure to respond." That's all you need to do — there's no need to find solutions right now. You'll discover plenty of those in the days to come. Simply by naming your sources of stress and how they affect you, you will find more relief and inner spaciousness.

Take Claire, for example. She's married, raising a three-year-old, building a business, seeing clients, and running her family's household. She often stays up until 2:00 or 3:00 in the morning to get her work done after her family has gone to sleep, only to wake up a few hours later to the cries of her little girl. Mentally foggy and physically exhausted, she's too tired to exercise and instead turns to coffee and sugar to keep her going. Her hormones get out of whack, she gains weight, she feels ashamed of and disconnected from her body, and her mood swings intensify. All these things cause a riff in her marriage. She's stuck in an endless cycle of trying to do so much for others that she has no energy to take care of herself and each day grows more angry, depressed, depleted, and resentful. Sound familiar?

Like Claire, we can feel controlled by our minds and are often afraid of our feelings. We manipulate, coerce, and curse our bodies until we break down. For some women, this struggle looks extreme; for others it's a subtle inner battle of vague discontent. But it doesn't have to be this way. We can take our health

THE POWER OF JOURNALING

My journals have been some of my best friends during the past two decades. Stacks of them reside in my home, and each one chronicles major milestones in my life: my first love, my first heartbreak, my first year in college, dips into depressions, euphoric expansions, new homes, world travel, and so much more. Writing in my journal has been a crucial means of developing an intimate trust in my inner wisdom and an outlet to freely process uncensored emotional distress that otherwise I would have held captive in my body.

Even when you're not going through extreme life changes, journaling offers a useful way to examine the intersection between your inner and outer worlds daily. This process can't just happen mentally. A transformation occurs when you meet the page with your pen and your words flow. A wise witness emerges from within you — the one who can extract the insights and magic from whatever you're presently living through and help you to see how to apply them. Here resides an important ingredient in reclaiming your creativity. I found the courage to write this book only after doing Julia Cameron's twelve-week creativity recovery plan, as described in *The Artist's Way*, and committed to write at least three handwritten pages in my journal each day. When you journal, even if it's just a page before bed each night, a deeper part of you can come forth and share her voice. She's not your mind. She's your soul. And she holds the key to your truest happiness.

Dr. Christiane Northrup, women's health pioneer and author of *Women's Bodies, Women's Wisdom* and *The Secret Pleasures of Menopause*, advocates regular journaling and employs it with thousands of women in their journeys to greater health and happiness in all stages of life. Since emotional distress rests at the root of most women's physical and psychological ailments, no woman can afford to live without this simple yet tremendously potent self-reflective tool.

You do need a journal for this journey we'll take together. If you don't have one, take a trip to your favorite stationery store to buy a journal that reflects you. It doesn't have to be fancy: I usually spend less than four dollars on mine and get simple spiral-bound notebooks with colors and designs that appeal to me. Write your name inside, and add the date too, since it's fun to go back years (or even a few months) later and marvel at how much you've grown.

and happiness into our own hands simply by remembering who we truly are — deeply intuitive, spiritual beings intimately connected to the rhythms and cycles of nature. And the first step is simply to look inside and welcome what you find there.

To help get you started, here are a few examples of topics you can write about in your journal:

- The three possible times during my day when I'm likely to have twenty to thirty minutes to write in my journal are:
- Some things that are on my mind right now that I haven't had the time or space to talk to anyone about are:
- Out of those things, the one I'm feeling most called to explore in my journal right now is:
- The three main emotions that I feel about this situation, and where I feel those in my body, are [Example: "I feel fear in my belly."]:
- Two concrete ways that I can better support myself with this include [Example: "To take a time-out, lie on my back, place my hands on my belly, and take some deep breaths."]:

YOU ARE NOT ALONE

The more you connect with yourself in meaningful ways, such as journaling, the more you'll realize one of life's most basic, beautiful truths: we are *all* connected. But even more, we really do need one another. When we live in hurried isolation we deny the feminine values that heal and inspire us: connection, collaboration, inclusiveness, nurturance, generosity, expressiveness, and playfulness. According to Louann Brizendine, author of *The Female Brain*, after only eight weeks in utero, the neurons in our brains morph to generate these qualities by developing the areas that govern communication and emotion (while the neurons in male brains concentrate more on the areas of sex and aggression).[1]

When you dare to make a deeper connection with yourself and other women, you play a pivotal role in resuscitating the medicine of feminine wisdom in your family, your community, and your world.

Helen came to one of my red tent mini-retreats a few years ago. These red tents are three-hour women's yoga and meditation retreats to offer solace, rest, insight, and community in the midst of our busy lives. A successful businesswoman, Helen spends a lot of time traveling, leading high-powered meetings, and sealing top-dollar deals. She started coming to the red tent retreats because she was tired of always being in control and longed to reconnect with her femininity. On retreat, she sat in a circle of women and could finally feel safe enough to let down her guard. When she did, tears spilled down her cheeks. She felt such relief at being able to relax into her softness and the vulnerability that came from telling people the truth about how she felt. Finally, she could reveal her deep need and desire to feel supported and received for who she is, rather than for what she does.

Ask yourself: What do I need help with right now? What are my basic needs each day? What do I have to do to keep my life functioning? What do I need to do to keep my spirit alive? How much sleep do I need to feel good? How much alone time? What foods make me feel good? What activities truly energize and inspire me? What brings me bliss?

Then ask: How many of these needs can I realistically meet on my own? Who can I ask to help me with the rest? A girlfriend, spouse, family member,

FIGHT OR FLIGHT VS. TEND AND BEFRIEND

Our nervous systems function on two different levels — sympathetic, or "fight or flight," and parasympathetic, or "tend and befriend." Every woman needs to know how to move from the former to the latter, regularly. Quickened breathing, pulse, and heart rates, cued by the rapid release of the stress hormones, characterize the sympathetic response. When we live on adrenaline our bodies go berserk: hormones get out of whack, metabolism slows, sleep gets erratic, blood sugar levels go haywire, and moods swing. This is the stressful state most of us live in today and from which disease grows.

However, when the parasympathetic response, also known as "rest and digest," kicks in, the exact opposite — healing — happens. Your respiratory and heart rates slow down, circulation returns to the organs in the core of the body (which helps digestion), and your whole system finds a sense of ease. Ideally, we'd live from this place most of the time — until we encountered a serious threat that required us to take action. Our bodies find their innate equilibrium when they're in the parasympathetic mode and feel-good hormones such as oxytocin (most often associated with inducing uterine contractions, the letdown of milk, and mother-infant bonding during the birth process) flood through us.

Nicknamed "the love hormone," oxytocin offers benefits that extend far beyond childbirth. Many of the health benefits we associate with everyday pleasurable experiences and strong social connections start with oxytocin, for it decreases stress hormones and helps lower blood pressure. Oxytocin is released in the brain even in response to engaging in any activity that brings you joy and to hugging, kissing, and simple touching like holding someone's hand.[2]

The benefits of the love hormone in women continue to be discovered. A UCLA study revealed that when women are under stress and gather for support, the tend-and-befriend response kicks in and oxytocin is secreted, helping to curb the fight-or-flight response.[3] In short, science now supports what girlfriends have always known. We need one another.

Every day, as much as possible, encourage the release of oxytocin in your body through connecting with others and doing things that bring you pleasure, for embodied delight is one of the most potent medicines you can give yourself.

coach, therapist, neighbor, masseuse, coworker, employee? One of the best ways to plug into an instant support system is through joining or starting a women's circle. For millennia women's circles have been safe, nonjudgmental havens. In these circles women gather together to create, celebrate, grieve, and grow. If you're not already part of such a group, you can visit www.The WayoftheHappyWoman.com to find a group near you, join our online Virtual Women's Circle, or learn how to start one.

As women, we're hardwired to gather and to "tend and befriend." So this year (and the next and the next), try reaching out. See what happens when you stop being the giver all the time. Ask for help. Receive it! *You are not alone.*

REDEFINING HEALTH, HAPPINESS, AND BALANCE

We all have certain feelings, body parts, or aspects of our lives that are uncomfortable to face. But it's in turning toward, rather than away from, what we most fear that we come alive and own our true power. And that's what this is all about: being present for what's right in front of you, as if it's the most important thing in the world — because it *is*. When you do this, even if you're sick or disabled, you can still be healthy because you're living in alignment with the way things are. Living in such a way generates an inner glow that's infectious. My grandmother, who died at the age of ninety-one, lived this way. She hardly ever exercised or ate anything green, but she exuded an inner light and childlike joy because she was gratified by her life and was always surrounded by people she loved. Envision someone you know who exercises every day, eats only organic foods, and has a to-die-for wardrobe but who sulks and never smiles. Sure, outer habits do matter a great deal, but ultimately health's an *inner* state of being. It's the ability to be with yourself and with whatever life brings you. It's having an openhearted presence and a willingness to trust that whatever's in the way *is* the Way.

Another word for the kind of happiness I am describing is *contentment*. It's about being at ease with life's highs *and* lows. It's broadening your spectrum of feeling. Instead of playing it safe in the land of monotonous gray, you're engaging the whole rainbow of emotions, from red to purple, by trusting that everything you're experiencing will change, and, that, through it all, *you will be okay*. When you let happiness be an overall state of being that doesn't depend on your moods or your circumstances, you empower yourself to find the good in every situation. Each bump on your path provides an opportunity to discover your true happiness. Think about the major crises in your life. What gifts did they bring you? Now, reflect on some smaller mishaps from earlier today or this week (you broke your favorite dish, got in a fight with your partner, or spilled coffee on your blouse). Even those mishaps hold lessons for you when you're willing to look (how to let go of things you love, how to do what's right without needing to be right, and how to not take yourself so seriously). Those lessons are the building blocks for lasting happiness.

Even if you don't consider yourself a "happy person," that can change (take it from someone whose childhood heroines were Sylvia Plath and Anne Frank!). A daily focus on what we're grateful for, on what's working, and on pleasure-inducing activities (sleeping and eating well, exercising, relating with others, having sex), can help change your happiness set point. But it takes effort. There's nothing spontaneous and magical about happiness. You have to develop it, participate in it, and knead it like bread in order to feast on it.

Last, you need to think about balance differently. And by balance I don't mean deftly juggling all the balls in your life — relationships, career, family, health, finances, spirituality — without fumbling or dropping any of them. That kind of balance is a fallacy. Instead, I mean two things: slowing down and synchronizing with nature's rhythms to restore your inner state of homeostasis and getting clear about your main priorities and structuring your life accordingly.

When we get out of our own way, our bodies know how to bring us back to homeostasis. They want us to be at the right temperature, to have the right amount of energy depending on the time of day, the season of the year, or the stage of life. They want us to have the right amount of water, fire, earth, and air in our cellular makeup. They want us to stretch toward the light, to grow, to evolve. The planet and all her creatures also know about balance, about thriving on a divine equilibrium between all the elements. In this book I hope to show you how to align with that primordial balance.

The second definition calls you to get realistic about what's going on in your life and to home in on what you value most. Maybe you've had a baby, or you're launching a new business, or you're about to move to a new city. These things are all part of life, and we don't need to berate ourselves for being out of balance when we let our exercise regime slide or we're eating more pizza than usual because we don't have time to cook during these transitions. In the short term, sometimes we do need to put some things on the back burner for the sake of a larger purpose. True balance is about being a warrioress when it comes to what matters to you most and being gentle with yourself when life throws you a curve ball. This kind of balance calls for clarity, adaptability, and flexibility.

SELF-CARE ISN'T SELFISH

Whether or not we realize it, most of us women were raised to put our needs second to those of others. However, you have nothing to give if your tank's on empty. You need to fill yourself up first before offering some of your overflow to others. If you don't, you're on the fast track to burnout and resentment. Ask yourself this: If your mother had taken better care of herself, would you have had a better childhood? Most likely, your answer is a resounding yes! Modeling self-care for your children is one of the most valuable gifts you can give them. You're demonstrating a crucial component of staying happy and healthy as an adult. Just as on an airplane when the adults are instructed to put on their oxygen masks before helping their children, we need to meet our own needs first before trying to meet the needs of others.

> ### TRY THIS
>
> In your journal, on the far-left side of the page, make a list of all the roles you play (mother, sister, boss, wife, daughter, friend). Be sure to leave a few lines after each role. Then, next to each one, list all the responsibilities you have in that role. When you've finished, number the roles from most important to least important. Using a highlighter or a colored pencil, circle the top three roles to remind you where your heart most wants to focus when you start getting pulled in too many directions.
>
> Did you include your relationship to yourself on that list? If not, that's about to change. *Always* put yourself at the very top of your priority list.

One of my yoga and meditation teachers, Sarah Powers, travels around the world teaching with her husband while homeschooling her daughter. It sounds like a frazzling lifestyle, and it would be if she didn't partake in daily yoga and meditation practices and go on a handful of retreats each year. She and her husband take turns going away. They see it as crucial for their growth, for staying happy and fulfilled, and for modeling for their daughter how to be sane adults. In your life, what do you really need or want but have been putting off because you think it's selfish? Is it to take time to get some exercise every day? To get a babysitter so you can have an afternoon to yourself? To treat yourself to a pedicure every month, buy yourself flowers, or go away with some girlfriends for a weekend? Maybe it's to hand over one of the middle-of-the-night feedings to your partner so you can catch up on sleep. Go ahead! I give you full permission to take excellent care of yourself and to be "selfish"!

TELLING YOUR STORY

One winter I led a women's yoga class in Chiang Mai, Thailand. To start off, we sat in a big circle, and I asked each woman to introduce herself, share how she was feeling in that moment, and tell us what she needed to receive from the group that day. One of my longtime students, Monica, had scrambled in late and was hiding on the outskirts of the circle near the door. When it was her turn to share, I invited her to take a seat in the circle and take a few deep breaths to really "land" before she spoke. I knew that Monica had been going through a lot — navigating a rough patch in her marriage while raising two young boys and growing her career.

TRY THIS

In your journal, tell your story by completing the following sentences. If you're an experienced journal writer, feel free to morph these into paragraphs and to write as much as you'd like.

1. Looking back on my life, I'd say that the five main events — good and bad — that have really formed who I am include:
2. Out of these, I planned __ of them, and the other __ were unexpected.
3. The three biggest lessons that I've learned in my life from these events include:
4. Two things that I love most about my life right now are:
5. Two things that I would most like to change about my life right now are:
6. Two things that I'm ready to invite and receive into my life right now are:
7. Some of my goals and dreams that seem a little crazy and that I'm almost too embarrassed to admit are to:

When you're finished, choose a quiet time when you know you'll have privacy. Go into the bathroom and lock the door, perhaps once the kids have gone to sleep. Light a candle, and sit in front of a mirror. Reread what you've written to yourself. Speak your story and receive your truth. Look into your own eyes and really see yourself. When you're finished, honor yourself in some way. I like to put my hands together in front of my heart in *Namaste* position (*Namaste* is a Sanskrit word meaning "the light in me bows to the light in you") and gently bow to myself. Sometimes I smile and say, "I love you, Sara." Then simply notice how you feel, and leave a few minutes of space and silence before carrying on with your day or evening.

My own true happiness only came to me when I embraced everything about my reality, especially the parts that I didn't want to confess, much less own. You are no different. Take an honest look at everything you're feeling and experiencing. See it. Welcome it. Don't turn away from it. Start to get comfortable with being uncomfortable. Take a deep breath, and trust that you have the capacity to hold it all. Most likely your story contains ebbs and flows: times when you felt vibrant, confident, and active and times when you felt defeated and unsure, when all of a sudden you no longer recognized yourself or your life after some big changes. These cycles live in all our stories, in both big and little ways. Let's take a closer look at those cycles now.

Monica kept her tired eyes on the empty space in the center of the circle, her shoulders hunched forward. "I'm here because I knew I had to come," she said, her voice and her body beginning to tremble. "And, to be honest, I really don't know what I need right now. I guess I just need to know that I can be here as I am without needing to give anything to anyone. I'm just so tired." As her voice trailed off, tears began rolling down her cheeks. Everyone in the circle started to breathe more deeply because of Monica's courage in uttering a truth that each woman knew intimately in her own heart and life.

Throughout the class I watched Monica move through the practice, embodying a raw tenderness, elegance, and openness. Ironically, Monica, who is a physically strong woman, looked more powerful than ever that day in her surrender to her own brokenness.

REMEMBER

- Identify the main sources of stress in your life and how they affect you.
- You don't have to do this alone. Feel supported by the words of this book. Acknowledge anyone or anything in your life that nourishes you and your journey.
- Dust off (or buy) a journal. Write in it regularly to become more intimate with yourself and to befriend the voice of your wisdom, your soul.
- Practice the art of receiving. Figure out what you need help with, and ask for it.
- What balls are you juggling? Which ones are most important to you right now? Can you give yourself permission to focus on just those for a while?
- Take care of yourself first. There's nothing selfish about self-care.
- Know your story. Write it down. Acknowledge what has brought you to this place. Celebrate it, and share it with others.

Chapter 2

THE CYCLES THAT HEAL

I've spent almost every summer of my life on the sandy shores of Lake Michigan. In my late grandparents' cottage, perched right at the water's edge, I'm lulled to sleep each night by the sound of the waves. I always wake up rested — so rested, in fact, that it's often hard for me to part with such a deep slumber and enter the next day. When I return home from my visit, I always have a hard time falling asleep for the first few nights. I miss the waves. Each year I'm reminded of this fact: rhythm is deeply restorative. As babies we love to be rocked, and even as adults we're soothed by rocking chairs, porch swings, and slow dancing. Conversely, the cacophony of leaf blowers, car horns, and jackhammers jars our nervous systems, scrambles our rhythms, and dispels our ease.

Modern living has one tempo only — fast. We're expected to exert ourselves in the same way, at the same time, five days a week and to take rest only on weekends and holidays. This rhythm is in fact not a rhythm at all. It's a monotone — that is, until you crash. A more organic tempo stirs in human bodies and souls and in the earth herself — one that needs times to ease into things, to go full throttle, and then to rest. Women's moods and energy levels wax and wane like the moon, ebb and flow like the tides, flourish and decay like the seasons. Living in harmony with these cycles strengthens us, makes us wiser, and heals us. Denying them weakens our spirits, our bodies, and our connection to life herself.

What if you pulled away from this constant stimulation? Stepped out of this forward-gushing wave of modern life and did something else? What if you found your own rhythm, one that's insightful and nurturing like the lapping of waves on a sandy shore — sometimes rough, sometimes quiet, sometimes still like glass? Maybe you're afraid that you couldn't possibly get everything done if you weren't on the go all the time. Or you're afraid that you'd miss out on a great opportunity or let others down. I hear you. But you can't afford not to take the risk.

Within each of us lives this rhythmical spirit of the wild feminine — the woman who walks the earth like a barefoot queen, wearing the robes of wisdom, clarity, ferocity, and tender connection. She's waiting to be seen, felt, and expressed. The only way to resuscitate your inner wild woman is to feast on nature's cycles once again; for Mother Nature *is* another name for the Divine Feminine. You can feel and know her for yourself each time you are deeply fed by the light of the full moon, the dark quiet of a winter snowstorm, or the sound of raindrops on your roof.

SLOW DOWN AND PAY ATTENTION

Another way we can honor Mother Nature is to align with her cycles, for we always have two options — ignoring these cycles or participating with them. Unfortunately, most of us are too busy to notice these cycles. Participating with them requires learning how to pause and pay attention to the constant changes in our bodies and surroundings.

When I started menstruating at the age of thirteen, instead of being taught how to honor this rite of passage, I was simply instructed to pop in a tampon. In fact, I even wore my new pair of tight, white jeans that day and inwardly applauded myself for not staining them! That was the sum total of my celebration that day. But when we live in harmony

---

TRY THIS

Here are some simple ways to connect with Mother Nature, even in a big city or during a busy day:

1. Before you get out of bed in the morning, look out your window. Take three to seven full breaths. Inhale the colors, shapes, and textures around you. Don't think about it — just breathe it all in, even if it's just a patch of sky. Notice how you feel.

2. As you walk to and from your car (or from building to building), feel your feet on the ground. Imagine that your mind is in your feet — feel them there completely. Notice your weight as it shifts from heel to ball, foot to foot. Any time you notice yourself thinking, just note to yourself "thinking" and return to feeling your feet on the ground.

3. Give yourself permission to mimic the weather with your mood. If it's raining or snowing outside, let yourself be lazy on your couch or a little bit contemplative and melancholy, if that's how you're feeling.

4. Bring nature indoors. Open the window. Buy some houseplants. Don't be afraid to talk to them (or to listen to what they have to say to you). Keep a vase of fresh flowers on your kitchen table. Start an indoor herb garden. Put a crystal on your desk or a small fountain in the corner of your living room. Find ways to bring the colors and vibrancy of the natural world into your home.

with our cycles, honoring the quiet valleys and the expressive peaks, our intimacy with ourselves and with all of life deepens. The weather and the length of the day become the portal through which we feel our aliveness. But let's be realistic: living in sync with nature is both the easiest and most natural thing we could do and one of the most challenging. It's challenging because it means going against the flow by taking the time to slow down, letting your body lead the way, making outdoor activities a priority, and spending the time and money preparing food and beverages that truly nourish you. The world isn't going to slow down. But you can.

RETREATING

Retreating — the act of stepping out of life and into the recesses of your inner world — is a feminine act. A downbeat in our varied rhythms, it's the ultimate way to slow down and pay attention. Moreover, retreating is a necessity. Liz, mother of five, leaves the house and goes to a yoga class as a mini-retreat. Diane goes for a walk around a small lake near her home. Susan meditates each morning and lets her children crawl around her or snuggle up on her lap as she sits. Here are some other simple ways to retreat:

- Close the door to your office and hang up a Do Not Disturb sign. Lie down. Play soothing music, take off your shoes, and close your eyes. Place your hands on your belly, and breathe deeply into them.
- Transform a chore into a ritual. Choose something you do every day, such as brushing your teeth, drinking a glass of water, or washing the dishes. Shift your focus from your thoughts to what you're doing. Play some nice music and enjoy yourself.
- Curl up on the couch with your favorite blanket, a cup of tea, and a good book or magazine. Instead of returning that phone call or email, indulge in delight and comfort for fifteen (or more!) minutes.

HONORING THE SEASONS

As I'm writing this it's the last day of August here in Boulder, Colorado. The days are about ten degrees cooler now than they have been for most of the summer, and evening and early mornings feel like fall. These seasonal shifts are the most pronounced way that we experience cycles — for they affect what we wear, what we eat, and what activities we engage in. They even affect how we feel (we'll explore this topic in greater depth in parts 2 to 5).

Nature knows how to blossom, flourish, decay, dissolve, and be born again. This gives her stamina through renewal and beauty through change — things we embody when we too flow with the seasons. The more you participate in seasonal changes, the more powerfully they will work for you to move through your own larger stages of birth, growth, and dissolution. Throughout your life you move through spring in your childhood, summer in your adulthood, autumn in your late adulthood, and winter as you transition toward death.

Each month our bodies go through mini-seasons with our menstrual cycles. We're continually incubating, creating, shedding, and letting go. At ovulation we're ripe and fertile, much like the earth at the height of summer. The week

TAOISM AND NATURE'S CYCLES

In need of a healer when I first moved to Chiang Mai, I asked a friend for a referral, and he sent me to his beloved Traditional Chinese Medicine (TCM) doctor, Dr. Po. I remember the first day I stepped off the hot street that buzzed with a steady stream of motorbikes and into her cool, serene clinic. A fountain rippled in the corner. Soft bamboo flutes serenaded the quiet space. The earthy aroma of exotic herbs enveloped the room like an invisible cloud. Then I saw Dr. Po, who very quickly became my "Thai mother."

Reaching across her desk, she took my hands in hers and squeezed them, telling me how happy she was that I had come. She looked at my tongue and listened to my pulse, told me to slow down and eat more, and sent me away with a huge bag of herbal pellets and told me to come back next week. It wasn't just her herbs and acupuncture that helped me to heal, but also her love and her faith in my body's ability to find harmony again.

The medicinal offspring of Taoism, TCM classifies nature according to the five elements — wood, fire, earth, metal, and water. These form an interrelated wheel of life that, when functioning properly, creates equilibrium. Wood grows out of water; fire burns from wood; fire generates earth by transmuting matter to ash; earth supports metal by bringing the soil's minerals to the surface; metal infuses water with vitality; and water once again moistens wood.

Each of these five elements corresponds to a different season of the year, organ system, emotion, taste, and odor, and even a different color and body part. TCM postulates that these elements from the natural world live in our bodies, both in our organs and in unseen energetic pathways, or meridians, through which chi (or vital life force energy) moves to govern everything from making your hair grow to causing planets to spin in space. In your body, the harmony among these five elements, as well as the strength and flow of your chi, determines the quality of your health.

before menstruation we start to contract and turn inward, as we do in the fall. When we bleed it's an inner winter. We hole up alone (ideally) to dream and regenerate. After menstruation we're reborn as we are in the spring, having let go, rested, and purified.

Even if you live in a place where the four seasons are not as distinct as they are here in Colorado, they still affect you — and I can say this with authority, having spent nearly a decade in Thailand! As you read, think about the seasons, and locate which one you're in both creatively and hormonally. From now on, rather than letting the seasons be a picturesque backdrop to your day-to-day routines or a chance to spruce up your wardrobe, let them also become the portal to your own evolution.

DAILY CYCLES

Just as the earth moves in cycles — from the bursting forth of spring to the quiet recoiling of winter — each of our days follows a similar pattern with clear cycles of activity and rest, also known as circadian rhythms. Inner cycles linked to the earth's cycles of day and night, our circadian rhythms govern all our body's activities, through the secretion of hormones, during each twenty-four-hour period. To maintain the health of these biorhythms we need to live much like our ancestors did. We need fresh air, sun, seasonal foods, rest, activity, community, and clean air and water. We need to sleep when it's dark and wake up when it gets light. These activities strengthen our circadian rhythms — while overscheduling ourselves, working at night, and exerting ourselves during our moon cycles weaken them.

Whenever you're feeling out of sorts, one of the best ways to get back on track is to realign with your daily rituals because they restore your basic sleep/wake, rest/activity, focus/wander rhythms (I'll share more about these daily rituals later in this chapter). For instance, when I was overcoming anorexia, I had a really hard time getting on an eating schedule again. I was so used to skipping meals and eating as little as I could that the idea of eating three solid meals a day, not to mention snacks, was foreign to me. When I started studying Ayurveda, India's ancient healing science, I realized that a lot of my imbalances (anxiety, poor digestion, insomnia) could be improved simply by sticking to a schedule. This would ground me and allow my body to find a steady rhythm. I trusted this ancient wisdom enough to give it a try, so I started to eat a solid breakfast, lunch, and dinner, consisting of foods appropriate for my constitution (more on that in chapter 4), at around the same time each day. I started waking up, going to sleep, and doing my yoga and meditation practices around the same time each day. Since then my health — at every level — has improved radically.

LIVING IN RHYTHM ALL YEAR

The healthiest, most successful and fulfilled individuals I know have a morning ritual. These rituals ground you in what matters before the hustle and bustle of the day begins. Veronica in Singapore sets her alarm at 5:30 every morning to do a thirty to forty-five-minute yoga practice before her children and husband wake up. Julia savors a cup of coffee while writing in her journal.

Every woman must develop her own morning ritual. Take into account whom you live with, what time you like to wake up, and how much time you have and are willing to spend on this. In most cases having a morning ritual will involve waking up a bit earlier than usual. At the very least, set your alarm for ten minutes earlier than usual and sit in bed with your eyes closed, feeling your breath. What activities appeal to you that you might like to incorporate into a morning ritual? If you already have one, what is it? Is it working for you, or is it in need of a revamping?

The morning ritual is just one part of your daily rhythm, though. As you create your daily rhythms, remember to allow yourself enough time so you don't have to rush. This may take some trial and error, but start by testing out how long it takes you to do things in a way that feels spacious and doesn't elicit stress. For example, give yourself an hour to shower, dress, and make and eat breakfast so you don't find yourself rushing around and then gobbling down some toast on your way out the door. I know it might seem challenging or overwhelming to develop a structured daily rhythm, but try it out, and you'll most likely find that discipline can be tremendously self-empowering! Congratulate yourself for creating new, healthy habits, and celebrate each step you take as a supreme act of self-love and respect. Here are some ideas for you to consider:

- *Waking up.* Ideally, you'll wake up without an alarm sometime between 5:30 and 7:30 A.M. On most nights, you'll need eight to nine hours of sleep, but if you're really run down, you'll need ten to eleven. If you must use an alarm, do yourself a favor and invest in one that doesn't jolt your nervous system!

- *Setting the tone.* Before springing up and jumping into the shower or digressing into the details of your to-do list, pause, relax your body, and take three deep breaths. Set an intention: "Today, I will choose happiness" — no matter what happens during the day. I love reciting the words "i thank You God most for this amazing day," from a poem by E. E. Cummings.

- *Developing a morning routine.* Every day I laugh at myself a little because the regularity of my wake-up routine feels a lot like the movie *Groundhog Day*. But that's also what's so sweet about it! Go to the bathroom. Look in the mirror and say, "I love you, [insert your name]!" Then brush your teeth and scrape your tongue (an Ayurvedic prescription to help remove excess mucus from the body). Use a neti pot if you're sick or congested to clear out your sinuses and make breathing easier. Drink one or two glasses of warm water with lemon and make yourself some tea. I recommend either something herbal or green tea or maté, since the caffeine in these is easier on your body than that found in black tea or coffee. However, if you're a coffee-loving woman, make sure the coffee's organic, and limit it to one cup!

- *Staying off the Internet.* Don't start your day checking email, reading blogs, texting, or making phone calls. If you start off with self-care and reflection instead, you will step into your day with much more presence and positivity.

- *Meditating.* For ten minutes, sit with your eyes closed. Observe and feel your breath (more instructions on page 44).

- *Doing yoga or exercising.* Get into your body right away, and you'll feel juicier and more vital all day (more instructions coming in parts 2 to 5).

- *Bathing and dressing as a self-care ritual.* Brush your skin to increase lymphatic circulation (instructions on page 83); give yourself a massage with sesame oil (instructions on page 190); shower or take a bath. Adorn yourself in beautiful clothes for the day. Anoint yourself as the goddess that you are!

- *Making breakfast.* Prepare and eat a delicious breakfast — recipes coming in the following chapters!

- *Initiating your work/activity period.* Start your workday with the task that will bring you the most fruitful long-term results. Look at your to-do list and ask yourself, "What is most essential? What would bring the most lasting value? What would I most enjoy doing from my list?" Usually we're most alert and creative at this time of day, so use it to your advantage! Save emails, errands, and phone calls for later in the day when your mind's less alert.

- *Making lunch.* Lunch should be your largest meal of the day because your digestive powers are strongest between 10:00 A.M. and 2:00 P.M. After lunch, give yourself some unstructured downtime. Go for a walk. Take a little nap. Do some light reading or Internet surfing for pleasure.

- *Continuing your work/activity period.* Now is the time to get all your errands done, to return phone calls, or to answer emails.

- *Unwinding.* Use this time to transition from "doing" to "being." Do some gardening, go for a brisk walk, read on the porch, take a gentle yoga class, get together with friends, play with your children, or listen to relaxing music.

- *Making dinner.* Make dinner a smaller meal than lunch, and eat at least three hours before you go to sleep. This will ensure that you sleep more soundly and that your body has a chance to rejuvenate overnight.

- *Fitting in some downtime.* Step away from your work, the computer, and any disturbing television shows or movies after dinner. Get the TV out of your bedroom for good!

- *Planning the next day the night before.* Planning for the next day helps you to get it down on paper and out of your head so you're not sorting it all out when your head hits the pillow and you turn out the light.

- *Resolving questions.* If there are any looming questions, things that are really on your mind, write them down. Here are some examples: "Am I supposed to sign up for that course that starts next week?" "How can I find new and creative ways to generate some income?" "How should I resolve this conflict with Maria?" When you ask a question like that, it allows your conscious mind to relax and your subconscious mind to take over in your dream world. Many times you'll wake up just knowing what to do. With bigger questions, you might need to ask more than once, so be patient.

- *Creating a bedtime ritual.* Now is when it's a good idea to set your alarm. Set it for an hour before your bedtime so you're reminded to stop whatever you're doing and take the time to prepare for sleep. Take a bath with lavender. Make a cup of chamomile tea or warm organic milk (this can be rice or almond milk too) with nutmeg. Rub sesame oil on your feet and in your scalp. Read something inspiring. You can also write two to three pages in your journal, including making a list of five or more things about your day that you feel grateful for. These can be as simple as "I am grateful for the ripe peach that I ate for lunch" or "I'm grateful for the feeling of happiness I had as I walked to work and smelled freshly cut grass."

- *Preparing your sleeping sanctuary.* Make your room as dark as possible when you sleep. If you need to, install shades, curtains, or blackout blinds on your windows. Unplug any electrical devices that might beep or flash. Make your bedroom your sanctuary. The darker and quieter it is, the more rested you will feel when you are in bed, and, ultimately, the better you will sleep.

- *Turning the lights off.* Go to sleep sometime between 10:00 and 11:00 P.M. After that you get an upward spike in your energy, and you might find yourself up until the wee hours of the morning, causing you to miss out on the important regenerative sleep that your organs need.

For those who are new to these ideas, choose one thing that really calls to you from the above list and start incorporating it into your life. Do this each day for the next thirty days. If you're more experienced, choose two or three things that you're not already doing, and if you're well versed in this kind of living, see how much you can align each day with a rhythm that feels wholesome and balancing to both your inner and outer worlds.

WHERE DOES YOUR TIME GO?

I know what you're thinking. I already have so much to do. How can I possibly make time to do more? I thought this was about doing less! I hear you, and I know it can seem like a lot at first. But it's not impossible. You need to stop doing one thing to make room for something else. So starting now, see how you're actually using your time. For one week — or 168 hours — track how much time you spend doing things. To help with this, use the time-tracker sheet found at www.My168hours.com. You can also use an online time tracker tool like www.Toggl.com. Eliminating activities that drain your energy and distract you from what you care about will help you make more time for taking care of yourself and for making the practices in this book a part of your life. Cut out fifteen or thirty minutes of Web surfing or TV watching to meditate and write in your journal.

YOUR MOON TIME

During certain times of each month, you will need to adapt these daily rituals because every twenty-eight to thirty days, your body and emotions move through each of the four seasons in lesser degrees as part of your natural hormonal cycle. These monthly mini-seasons correspond with what phase the moon is in and, in turn, your menstrual cycle, which I refer to in this book mostly as your "moon time" (since it mirrors the lunar cycle). There are thirteen lunar months a year, and most women menstruate about that many times annually as well. Each cycle lasts approximately 29.5 days, give or take a few days at either end. Just as the tides of the massive oceans ebb and flow in accordance with the cycle of the moon, so too do the fluids of your body. Each month, through our menstrual cycle, we have the opportunity to grow and dissolve and remerge again, just like the seas and the moon.

How well you take care of yourself each day will show up in the ease or dis-ease of your moon time — and, in time, in how menopause affects you. Balance, which biologically derives from our hormonal balance, is our natural state. When women have PMS or menopausal symptoms such as hot flashes (which includes about 80 percent of women today, more than ever before), we are suffering from hormonal imbalance, a diversion from our natural state that's entirely induced by stress, lifestyle, and emotions that have not been tended to. The remedy lies in becoming educated about the wisdom inherent in your monthly cycles and being willing to honor these fluctuations by taking pause regularly. Women simply can't claim true health and harmony if they ignore their monthly cycles and the underlying causes of their imbalance.

One of my greatest inspirations in restoring the rhythm of my menstrual cycle was Maya Tiwari. A maven in New York City's fashion world, she left it all behind for solitude, prayer, and rest in Nepal's Himalayas after she received a diagnosis of ovarian cancer. There, she dove into the healing traditions of her East Indian ancestors, including Ayurvedic cooking, yoga, meditation, and aligning with the lunar cycle. Not only did she heal herself in this way, but she has also gone on to become a healer for thousands of women around the world, including me. In her book *Ayurveda: Secrets of Healing*, she explains that when the menstrual cycle has not been affected by the use of contraceptive pills, harmful foods, or other disruptive activities, it remains in harmony with the cycles of the moon. Tiwari advocates clearing up any problems with your menstrual cycle, reproductive system, or general health simply by getting your cycle back onto this schedule.[1]

I cannot stress enough how imperative it is for women to heal their relationships with their menstrual cycles. I continue to meet women around the world who have no idea 1) what phase the moon is in, 2) that the moon bears any relation to their menstrual cycle, 3) how to realign their bodies with lunar rhythms, or 4) that they need to live any differently during their moon time than they do at other times of the month.

When my own menses began, I'd get cramps and have irregular cycles — not really giving much thought to them — until, in my late teens, some friends told me that the pill could help regulate my cycle. So I took it for a while, since everyone else seemed to be taking it, until something in me said, "This isn't right." Several months later I found myself in Thailand, starting to learn the larger lessons of my menses — what it is, how to care for myself during it, and what the tremendous power of this time of the month actually holds. I remember, after so many years of skipping a month or two of bleeding, or, during the height of my eating disorders, not menstruating for several months on end, the day in Thailand when "my moon" (which I like to call it now to honor my body's connection to the moon) finally returned. I felt her warm, distinct arrival and stopped what I was doing to quietly whisper "thank you" to my body for refinding her balance as an embodied woman.

Now, when strong emotions arise the week before my menses, I take notice. I know that these arise to communicate powerful messages about what's not working in my life and how I have fallen out of balance the previous month. I use this premenstrual week to slow down and become more internal. Then, when my menses begins, I withdraw from most activities and rest. If you work full-time and/or have children, take a stand for yourself and call in sick the first day of your cycle. Hire a babysitter, or ask your partner to take over childcare duties that day. This is protocol for many Asian cultures and an incredibly important monthly pause that has been lost. To make a shift, women must lead the way and educate men, children, other women, and employers of the importance of this time. The more we participate in the moon's rhythm, the more the blueprint of our hormonal cycles — and our trust in them — can be restored. To help you honor and partake in this rhythm, in each season, I offer specific practices to do to honor your moon time, as well as yoga practices (one for the full moon, one for the new).

TRY THIS

FULL MOON REFLECTIONS

The full moon represents fertility, celebration, completion, and fullness. During the three days of the full moon, choose healthy foods that signify deep nourishment to you. Bake bread, make nutritious desserts, and cook pasta, soups, and stews. Invite friends over for a candlelit dinner party. Go dancing. Slip into a hot bath laced with rose petals or rose essential oil. Get a massage or a facial. Take a vigorous yoga class. Stay up late, absorbed in a creative project. Take a moonlit hike or

(continued on next page)

FULL MOON REFLECTIONS *(continued)*

walk (even if it's just around your city block). Sit outside and take a "moon bath" — either clothed or, if you have the privacy and it's warm enough, in the nude. Leave a glass jar filled with pure water outside in the moonlight, and drink this healing nectar the next day. Often we have trouble sleeping during the full moon because our energy is heightened and our thoughts and emotions feel more pronounced. Use this extra energy for celebration, connecting with others, and generally being more social and outgoing.

In your journal, set aside twenty to thirty minutes on each full moon eve and contemplate the following:

1. What has arrived, departed, or transpired since the last full moon that wants to be celebrated right now?
2. What have I completed or achieved in the past month? In what ways am I proud of myself?
3. How would I most enjoy celebrating right now? (This can be as simple as lighting a candle and slipping into a bubble bath or inviting friends over for a potluck.)

NEW MOON REFLECTIONS

New moons represent rest, letting go, and planting new seeds. Ideally this is the time of menstruation, but even if your moon cycle isn't synced up with the lunar calendar, you can still use the three days of the dark moon to relax, sleep in, meditate, or curl up with a book. This is a good time to cleanse by eating simple foods such as fresh juices, fruits, salads, easy-to-digest comfort foods, eggs (during your moon time), simple soups, and steamed vegetables. Write down on a piece of paper the things that you're letting go of, and have a letting-go ceremony by burning the paper, either alone or with other women. Then write down or speak aloud what you're inviting in and wishing to create during the next month.

In your journal, set aside twenty to thirty minutes on each new moon eve and contemplate the following:

1. What seeds do I want to consciously plant, with love and patience, for this next cycle?
2. How can I more deeply rest, restore, and let go right now?
3. Are there any ways in which I'm afraid of or resistant to being alone right now? What would allow me to feel safer and more comfortable with solitude and silence?
4. What wisdom have I gleaned from feeling the darkness of difficult emotions? And from this what can I bring forth and share with my family, friends, and community to the benefit of all?

REMEMBER

- Find simple ways every day to connect with the outdoors.
- Give yourself permission to feel the mood and energy that each weather pattern, and each season, brings.
- Establish your daily rituals, especially your morning ritual. Decide what you're going to realistically incorporate, and stick to it for the next thirty days. Celebrate on the full moon, and rest on the new moon.
- View menstruation as a time to rest, reflect, and hone your wisdom and insight to purify, and elicit powerful changes in, yourself and your community.

Chapter 3

A WOMAN'S INNER WORLD
Yoga and Meditation

When was the last time you woke up and asked your-self, "What am I feeling now, and what are these emotions try-ing to tell me?" or "What do I need to do to nourish my spirit today?" Most likely these weren't the first thoughts to pop into your head this morning — or any morning, for that matter. Even pondering them might conjure a big blank. However, one of the greatest gifts you can give yourself is to become adept in the language of your inner world by checking in with your feelings and then honoring them by acting from what you discover there. This is leading your life the feminine way — from the inside out.

Like a flower, your life can be divided into two parts: your inner world, the center of the flower, and your outer world, the petals. Your inner world consists of your thoughts, deepest heart's desires, intuitive knowing, awareness, devo-tion, and emotions. Your outer world includes your relationships, community, career, external personality, and day-to-day interactions. For the petals of your outer world to unfurl, you must first inhabit the innermost aspects of yourself — the bright and confident as well as the deflated and wounded parts. Doing so allows for authenticity, self-acceptance, self-love, trust, and confidence to flow into the outermost reaches of your life. When you live from the inside out you don't need the love and approval of others to feel worthy. You don't need ev-eryone to agree with you to feel successful. You're sure of who you are, for you're guided by a steady, unwavering inner stream of wisdom. When you live this way, you are aligned with what you value most, which gives you the stabil-ity to flow through life without becoming derailed.

This inward-guided life only comes from ongoing practice. Daily, and even moment-to-moment, you must train yourself to check inside first before looking outside for direction. This takes time, discipline, and willingness, and every woman must determine for herself how much of those qualities she has at any given time. Above all, it takes courage and trust. Like any path, it grows more inviting each time it's walked on.

INTUITION

Albert Einstein once said, "The intuitive mind is a sacred gift and the rational mind is a faithful servant. We have created a society that honors the servant and has forgotten the gift."[1] Like a buried treasure, intuition awaits discovery at the heart of your inner world. It is the most essential ingredient in learning how to trust yourself and to lead a spirit-guided and heart-centered life. Unfortunately, in our world, just as your moon time is no longer honored, neither is your intuition. Certainly deep, inner listening isn't a skill we're taught in school or at home by our parents. But it's never too late to learn. In fact, our monthly cycles offer the perfect opportunity. During menstruation (or, for postmenopausal women, during the dark moon), when we retreat and step back from our worldly endeavors, we slow down, get quiet, and can then look inside and ask for guidance. At the end of our moon time, or as the sliver of a waxing moon reappears in the night sky, we can reenter our lives with new wisdom and fresh insight to implement our visions for positive change.

I've made two of the most pivotal decisions in my life based on intuition. The first was to move to Thailand. Then, nine years later, I knew I had come to the end of my time there. I had just left a five-year relationship, my sister was about to give birth to her first baby back in the States, and I felt a longing to be closer to my family and to move on to the next chapter of my life. Yet I felt torn inside. As a freelance writer and yoga teacher, I could live anywhere in the world. The options felt overwhelming. So I prayed for guidance, for a crystal-clear knowing of what my next step would be. And then I waited. A month later, I was in Rishikesh, India, just out of a ten-day meditation retreat. Standing on my yoga mat in mountain pose, I watched the sun rise from behind the mountains just outside my window. Suddenly, I felt a flash of light move through my body. Disoriented, for a moment I felt as if I was in Boulder, Colorado, where I had spent a lot of time in the past. Each time I had visited there, a small voice inside me whispered, "I'd love to live here one day." All of a sudden I just *knew* that now was the time to move there.

Intuition can come in many ways: through an inner vision, a dream, a bodily "feeling" or "knowing," a quiet inner voice, or external signs, coincidences, and synchronicities.

Here are a few simple ways to begin strengthening your intuition and getting to know how she best reveals herself to you:

- Throughout the day, ask as many times as you can, "What do You want me to do now?" (the "You" being your highest self, your deepest knowing, or the Divine). Start asking this about simple things — like which pair of earrings you should wear or what you should eat for breakfast. The more you ask the question, the more trained you will become in receiving answers, and you can start using this technique for bigger and bigger life decisions.

- Write in your journal with your nondominant hand. For me, that's my left hand. When I write with my right hand, I'm accessing the lineal, logical part of my brain. Try writing down a question with your dominant hand, such as "How should I handle this argument with my colleague?" and then pass your pen to your nondominant hand and see what answer comes out.

- Make a regular practice of telling life what you really want. You can do this in your journal, as a prayer before you go to sleep, or in a conversation with the sky as you go for a solitary walk. At the end of your request ask for clear, recognizable signs that you've been heard and that you will be shown the way. Then receive the symbols that show up — either in your dreams or through animals, numbers, or coincidences.

- Take time for a yoga, meditation, and journaling practice. This is when I get my best ideas!

- Spend time alone walking in nature, without your phone or iPod.

When I feel creatively stuck with my writing or work project, often a walk outside will infuse me with fresh insights.

> ## TRY THIS
>
> In your journal, make a list of all the times you can think of when your intuition spoke to you — when you just "had a feeling" about something. Include even the small moments, such as when you were thinking about your friend and she emailed you five minutes later. The more you become aware of these synchronicities, the more frequently they'll appear and the more profound they'll be.
>
> Now look back over that list. Are there any big events there? Times when your intuition bubbled up or a seemingly random coincidence significantly changed the course of your life in an unexpected way? If so, how did this turn out differently than a plan you might have concocted in your mind about your life's path?

THE POWER OF SILENCE

Silence is the container out of which your intuition can reveal herself. When your mind's racing, when the music is blaring, or when a garbage truck is barreling down the street, it's very hard to hear the subtle promptings of your inner wisdom. In a world where each moment can easily be filled with making phone calls, checking email, or sending text messages, short periods and, eventually, longer stretches of silence are imperative for cultivating a rich inner world.

Each winter during my annual women's retreat I inform students during our opening circle that we will observe silence every day from 9:00 P.M. to 9:00 A.M. and that for the duration of the retreat they are requested to relinquish their reading materials, stay off their computers and cell phones, and keep the TV and DVD players off. Although they've been told about this beforehand, I can still see the color drain from their faces when I share the morbid news! I know, I know: it can be terrifying to strip away the things that keep us busy and to face what's inside us. Open space is scary, and we want to fill it to find comfort. But once people actually do clear away distractions, they learn to fall in love with silence and spaciousness.

Silence recharges your batteries by stripping away the excess sensory stimulation from the outside world. It provides a container in which you can hear the voice of your soul. It's the medicine that most of the world needs right now — and fears.

Here are some ways to bring more sacred silence into your life:

- Spend the early-morning hours — until after breakfast — in silence. Don't check email, and turn off the ringer on your phone (and/or turn off your cell phone). If you live with others, get them on board, and practice relating to one another in a different way — through loving touch, notes, and glances.
- Eat one meal a day alone — without reading, listening to music, surfing the Web, or watching TV. If you have children, do it once a week or every other day. Alternatively, have a solo breakfast or lunch when the kids are at school or napping.
- Go on a technology fast one day a week. Stay away from your phone, computer, TV, iPod, even any sort of reading materials. Spend time outside, get out your art supplies, take a yoga class. Go for a bike ride, or have a picnic with your family. Sit outside and do absolutely nothing.
- Go on a silent retreat at least once a year.

- Have a silent retreat at home for one hour, half a day, a full day, or a week-end (I'll give you instructions on how to do this in parts 2 to 5).
- Set your phone so that calls automatically go to voice mail. Then choose when you want to call people back.

Ultimately silence becomes a serene stillness that you carry inside you — even as you cross the street in Times Square.

BARE ATTENTION

There are more ways to create space and silence, one being simply paying attention. Pretty straightforward, right? Well, yes and no. Living attentively, with awareness, day-to-day, moment-to-moment, takes real dedication and perseverance. It requires going against the grain from how we've become accustomed to living — floating around like bodyless heads, lost in nostalgia about the past or fantasies about the future. Instead, paying attention, or "bare attention," requires that you inhabit the present moment and simply notice what you find there, without trying to change, control, or escape it in any way. It infuses even the most ordinary of moments with sacred attention — so much so that I consider it one of my best friends and my most powerful spiritual practice.

Another name for this bare attention is mindfulness, a potent tool that you can use anytime, anywhere. It arrests the impulse to live on automatic pilot and brings you home, with vividness and intimacy, to the present moment. Dipa Ma, an Indian woman born in 1911 who became a revered Buddhist master, exemplifies how mindfulness can empower a woman. She lived in Burma with her husband and endured much suffering through the deaths of two of her children, her own frail health, and, later, the death of her husband. As is common for women in Southeast Asia, throughout all this she made frequent

> ### TRY THIS
>
> To sharpen your bare-attention skills, take a moment to put this book down (after you finish reading these instructions). Feel as much of your body as you can. Where do you notice tension? Ease? Without changing anything, just notice. Now, can you feel your breath? Where do you feel it in your body? Next, feel the surfaces that your body is touching. Look around you. What colors, shapes, and textures do you see? For example, as I sit at my desk here I see a puffy white cloud outside the window, I hear leaves blowing in the breeze, and on my desk I see a tall glass of water and a stack of books. Keep it simple, and don't go into a story about why things are the way they are (like "Oh, I really need to file that stack of papers"). Just notice.

trips to her local Buddhist temple to offer food to the monks and ask for bless-ings. During one visit, before her husband's passing, Dipa Ma voiced her long-ing to study meditation and was turned away. However, after her husband's death, when she was nearly drowning in her grief and growing frailer by the day, she went to the temple's meditation center and literally crawled up the stairs on her hands and knees to learn. This time, she wouldn't take no for an answer.

Ripe for uncovering a place of inner peace and happiness that lay beneath and beyond her suffering, Dipa Ma progressed quickly in her meditation stud-ies and soon reached very enlightened states. However, she didn't stay tucked away in the temple. She returned to her life as a householder, supplementing that life with regular retreat times to continue going deeper. Soon the women in her neighborhood heard about Dipa Ma's miraculous transformation from a frail, melancholy woman to a bright, strong, loving heroine. Wanting what she had, they came to her for teachings. Knowing the reality of these wom-en's lives as wives and mothers, Dipa Ma offered the most practical advice she could: Practice mindfulness. Feel the cloth as you fold your laundry and hang it on the line. Notice the temperature of the water on your skin as you wash the dishes. Sense your baby's lips on your breast as she feeds. Turn away from your thoughts and become present to moment-to-moment sensations as you do your daily chores. The women listened. They went back to their husbands, homes, and children and practiced mindfulness. Soon they too uncovered deeper truths about themselves. Their previously mundane tasks, when done with great pres-ence, brought them into the same deep states of all-pervasive awareness that many hours of meditation can bring about. Her story reminds us: No matter how busy you are, you can meditate each moment of your life just by being mindful.

BEING WITH YOUR EMOTIONS

Once we get grounded in mindfulness, we're more present to everything, in-cluding our emotions. If you're not equipped with the skills to be with your emotions in a wholesome way, this can cause problems. As women, our limbic systems are larger than those of men — meaning that we feel more, and more deeply. Depending on how you relate to them, these emotions can be either a blessing or a curse. Since most of us never received any real education in how to relate to our feelings, they have been more like a curse. They rock us. They can ruin our day and even sabotage relationships. As women we need to learn how to feel our emotions fully without getting pummeled by them.

Throughout each season of the year certain emotions will come on more strongly, such as anger in the spring and sadness in the fall. On a smaller scale, within a single day you can experience a few dozen different emotions (or more). You don't need to ignore them, and you don't need to be consumed by them, but you do need to find a healthy balance between acknowledging them, allowing them to be there, and feeling them. These emotions play a large role in the development of our intuition. For example, when emotions such as fear, anger, or sadness arise, these are messages from your body that it's time to make some changes. When emotions such as joy, gratitude, and love emerge, they're clear signals for you to continue on your present path.

Holding back tears because you're embarrassed to cry, eating a pint of ice cream in the middle of night to bury your loneliness, and feeling it's not "ladylike" to voice your anger are all examples of ignoring your emotions and preventing them from flowing. The same can be said for emotions such as joy and excitement.

> ## TRY THIS
>
> Reflect on the past twenty-four hours. Write down all the emotions you remember having felt. This list might include some of the big ones, such as anger, fear, joy, or sadness. But most likely it will hold more of the subtler ones, such as boredom, doubt, regret, satisfaction, dullness, enthusiasm, and confusion. Once you've compiled your list, look over it again. What do you notice? I hope that you will recognize your tremendous capacity to sound a whole range of notes — *and* will see that none of them lasts forever!

I remember being in the sauna at Kripalu, a yoga center in western Massachusetts, one evening during a yoga retreat. I was lying down in the yoga pose *virasana*, or Hero's Pose, and a strong feeling of pleasure — like a warm flow of golden honey — started moving up my thighs, pelvis, and belly. My first, unconscious impulse was to make it go away by changing positions. But I stopped myself. Mindfulness interrupted my habits of avoidance, and I stopped and got curious about what was going on. What was so uncomfortable about this? I realized that pleasure, although a positive experience, was also a strong feeling, accompanied by strong sensations. And I was afraid of feeling it. A lightbulb came on for me: It didn't matter whether a feeling was pleasurable or unpleasant; if it came on strong in my body, my first impulse was to lessen it or make it go away. That evening, however, I made a shift. I felt the pleasure fully.

THE ONLY WAY OUT IS IN AND THROUGH

How exactly does one develop this capacity to stay with strong emotions? With the DNA of hunters and warriors in our genes, we're hardwired to run from pain and cling to pleasure. However, true evolution and inner freedom come not from pushing and pulling reality according to our preferences but from stepping into the heart of what's directly in front of us — even if it's uncomfortable. If you're to remember one thing about your feelings, it's this: *The only way out is in and through.*

Running from your feelings, burying them, and sedating yourself in the face of them are all short-term fixes that do more harm than good. However, once you step into the mouth of whatever dragon confronts you, that dragon *will* eventually dissolve, releasing you, transformed and freer, from its grip. Sometimes this happens right away, and sometimes it happens over a long stretch of time (even years for really ingrained emotional patterns). But everything will and does change — it's a fundamental law of life that nothing stays the same.

Here's a simple formula to follow when you're confronted with a challenging emotion:

> ### TRY THIS
>
> One powerful way to feel your emotions in your body is through music and dance. I'm a firm believer that no woman should go more than a week without dancing! One exercise that always works for me is to make a playlist of several songs, each clearly eliciting a different mood and emotion (lightheartedness, rage, grief, sultriness) through its lyrics, instruments, tempo, and overall flavor. As you can imagine, some women feel more comfortable with this than others — and certainly every woman finds at least one of these emotions challenging to dance to. Here's a hint: whichever emotion scares you the most, that is the one that you need to dance to!

1. *Pay attention to it.* Use your mindfulness skills to come to the present moment. Step out of your thoughts and simply feel your body.
2. *Soften.* Let yourself relax rather than tensing up against what you're feeling.
3. *Name it.* "Oh, anger," or "Here's sadness again," or "There's fear."
4. *Locate the emotion in your body.* Is it in your belly? Chest? Throat? A combination of these?
5. *Explore the sensations.* Once you've located the feeling in your body, be curious about it. Is it hot or cold? Fluttering or solid? Does it move? If so, where and how?

6. *Stay with it*. When you notice yourself jumping back into your thoughts, keep returning to exploring the sensations in your body and how they change.

One of my students, Cathy, applied these steps to finally face her ongoing struggles with anxiety. When she came to Thailand a few years ago to participate in my teacher training course, anxiety attacks began to consume her midway through the training. Living in a community, as well as having to stand up as a teacher to lead her peers, caused her tendency toward panic attacks to surface. The familiar clamping down in her belly and throat, followed by an unsettled fluttering in her chest, plagued her.

I started by giving Cathy some simple instructions. Whenever she felt the anxiety coming on, she should sit or lie down in a comfortable place and get curious, like a scientist or a wonder-filled child. Then she should examine the sensations in her body — where did she feel them the most? In her belly, chest, throat? Did they stay there? Did they move? What temperature were they? Did they feel heavy or light? Fast or slow? Dense or airy?

I advised her, while asking these questions of her experience, to keep feeling the support underneath her and to stay connected with her breath, as she had learned to do during our mindfulness meditation practices. When thoughts or mental commentary surfaced, I told her to note them and to label them "thinking," and, afterward, to return to noting and feeling the sensations in her body.

These two tools — the clear, simple, and grounded practice of mindfulness and feeling and allowing the changing, flowing sensations in the body — form the bedrock of how we must learn to embrace our own fluid, ever-changing embodied aliveness as women.

MINDFULNESS MEDITATION

All these principles — intuition, silence, deep listening, bare attention, and locating where emotions live as sensations in the body — are refined in one practice: Mindfulness Meditation.

While it's not easy to carve out time for ourselves every day and, yes, some days we'd rather not sit in silence or move and stretch our bodies, these are essential ingredients for sanity! All you need is ten minutes. If you can manage more, great. I often tell people that I honestly don't think I'd be alive today if I hadn't learned yoga and meditation and if I didn't practice them regularly.

They've helped me process in a thorough and healthy way some of the deeply buried and most painful aspects of myself.

No matter how busy you are, do try to take a minimum of ten minutes a day to unplug and connect with yourself. I find that I'm most successful when I meditate first thing in the morning, before the world starts pulling me in all sorts of unexpected directions. Meditating just before bed can work well too.

Here's a simple yet powerful Mindfulness Meditation practice from the Buddhist tradition.

1. Sit in a chair so that your spine is long and your feet are flat on the ground (place some books, pillows, or yoga blocks underneath them if you need to). Or sit on the floor, cross-legged. If you're sitting on the floor, stack one or two blankets underneath your pelvis so that you're rocking on the front edges of your sitting bones and your hips are higher than your knees.

2. Set your timer for ten minutes, and commit to staying with your meditation practice that entire time — even if the phone or doorbell rings.

3. Rest your palms on your thighs.

4. Roll your shoulders up and back. Slide your shoulder blades down your back. Draw your chin in until your ears line up over your shoulders and your lower jaw is perpendicular to the floor.

5. Now, simply *relax* and *soften*. Release any tension from your face. Unfurrow your brow, slacken your jaw. Let go.

6. Arrive more fully in your seat. Feel your pelvis relaxing into the surface beneath you. Receive your breath in your belly. Let everything about your experience be simple; be curious about it all.

7. Now simply notice your breath. You can feel your breath flowing in and out of your nostrils, or you can notice your belly rise and fall with your breath. Choose one of these two places to focus your attention. Simply watch — and feel — your breath come and go.

8. Each time your mind drifts, come back to the anchor of your breath. You are simply sitting, breathing, noticing, and feeling. Anything else that comes into your awareness will no doubt be there waiting for you when you finish your meditation, if it's important enough.

9. At the end of your meditation, place your hands together in front of your heart in a prayer position. Gently bow in gratitude, wishing for your practice to be of benefit to all beings (yourself included!).

This practice will serve as the foundation for our meditation this year. Each season you'll learn additional meditations to cultivate your intrinsic heart qualities of loving-kindness, sympathetic joy, compassion, and equanimity.

Each season you'll also learn two new yoga practices — one for the full moon (or ovulation and creating) and the other one for the new moon (or menstruation and dissolving).

WOMEN'S YOGA

Yoga is a vast topic that has been written about extensively. Since so many good books go into detail on its history, various styles, philosophies, and practices, I won't go into these things in depth here. I will say that yoga is an immensely powerful and simple means of exercise, healing, self-discovery, and transformation. When practiced with curiosity and reverence it gives you the power to do so much, from strengthening your life force, overcoming internal and external obstacles, sleeping and digesting better, and maintaining a more balanced emotional and mental state to ultimately experiencing the essential truths and beauty of life — and yourself — with more presence and poignancy.

If you're brand-new to yoga, please find a teacher whom you enjoy at a yoga studio near you. If yoga's just not your thing, find out what is. But please do something — anything — physical each day for at least fifteen minutes. Stretch. Go for a walk around the block. Run. Jump rope. Use a hula hoop. Get on the elliptical machine at the gym. Swim. The key is not to ask too much of yourself. Start small so you'll succeed.

Since I first began practicing yoga in 1996 I have shifted from practicing and teaching a very masculine approach to yoga with the desire to perfect my body and control my life (by doing the same postures, in the same order, day in and day out, emphasizing form, and accomplishing advanced postures — regardless of how I was feeling) to a more feminine practice (one that is creative, intuitive, and honors how I'm feeling each day). While the first style of yoga cultivated a lot of strength, stability, flexibility, and technical prowess in my body and focus and discipline in my mind, it didn't help me to confront deeper wounds such as low self-esteem and poor body image and physical concerns such as weak digestion, insomnia, ovarian cysts, irregular menstruation, and anxiety. Only when I adapted a softer, more adaptive and intuitive approach to my practice could I start to heal at a deeper level and feel that I was truly

MENARCHE TO MENOPAUSE:
YOGA FOR THE CYCLES OF A WOMAN'S LIFE

Eighty to 90 percent of yoga classes are all female, yet very rarely do these classes teach women how to practice in a way that supports where they are in their monthly or life cycles. Here are a few basic guidelines to keep in mind when practicing yoga. If some of the yoga terms I use are foreign to you, not to worry: they'll be explained more in parts 2 to 5, or you can pick up just about any introductory yoga book (I've included a link to my favorites on my website).

PREMENSTRUAL YOGA

One week before your flow, start to slow down in every way. Do more hip openers, forward bends, deep breathing, and meditation to support your strong emotions and to prepare for the quiet time of menstruation. Try some restorative back bends if you're prone to breast tenderness, abdominal bloating, or cramping. If you tend to experience migraines, do inversions (but not when you have the headache), since these help balance your hormones. I offer a free one-hour audio *Yoga for PMS* CD on my website too (www.TheWayoftheHappyWoman.com).

MENSTRUAL YOGA

Do yin or restorative yoga on the first few days of your cycle. Avoid standing poses, inversions, and strong practices in general. Gentle chest openers can feel really nice too. Don't do any strong breathing practices or core strengthening. Your womb and belly need to feel relaxed and open to encourage the downward, purifying flow of your menstrual stream. Take more time for meditation to tap into the strong intuitive prompts that are available to you now.

POSTMENSTRUAL YOGA

Gradually start to intensify your practice again once your flow has ended. When your bleeding has completely stopped, start to invert again, since going upside down now helps to tone and strengthen your uterus. This is the time of month to focus on strength training and higher-intensity practices if you feel called to do so.

PRENATAL YOGA

Above all, listen to your body. She'll tell you what feels good and what doesn't. Your first trimester is a time to take it easy. Do more gentle practices, and join a prenatal yoga class for support and community. As your baby grows into the second trimester, you'll need to start modifying your practice. At a certain point, twists, abdominal crunches, deep back bends, inversions, and closed-leg forward bends feel uncomfortable and you'll need to omit or adapt these (a good teacher can show you how). During your final trimester, beware of putting too much pressure on your pelvic floor with a lot of standing poses. Find ways to deepen your connection to your baby, your breath, your inner meditative zone, and your overall state of relaxation to help you prepare for the marathon of labor and the miracle of motherhood.

POSTNATAL YOGA

Since every woman's birthing experience is different, each woman returns to her practice in her own way and time. Right after birth you can practice deep breathing, Final Relaxation pose, and pelvic floor exercises (or Kegels). Remember to really rest your body and to cherish the precious time with your little one for the first month. During your baby's naps in the early days you can do yin poses to help you rest and find yourself again. Chest and shoulder openers can feel especially good with all the breastfeeding and cradling you're doing. After you've stopped bleeding, supported inversions are wonderful (even just putting your legs up the wall when you're lying down in bed), as are long walks outside and a gradual reentry into your usual yoga practice, which is usually after six weeks if you've had a vaginal birth and eight weeks after a cesarean section. Please also work with a skilled yoga teacher and a pelvic floor physical therapist, if you can, to start strengthening and healing the muscles of your pelvic floor and abdomen to avoid organ prolapse, painful intercourse, or incontinence in the future.

MENOPAUSAL YOGA

Cooling, quieting practices will serve you now — especially during perimenopause and when you're in the throes of hot flashes and hormonal swings. Yin yoga, supported inversions, breathing practices, and meditation will help you harness your wisdom in this second half of your life. A slower, more mindful yoga practice will keep your body vital, while staying guided by your inner compass.

coming home to my feminine self. Ultimately each woman must develop her own organic relationship with herself to weave together the threads of her body, soul, and mind.

All of us, men and women alike, need a combination of masculine and feminine energies, both in our yoga and in our lives. Unfortunately, since we live in a male-oriented society, masculine qualities reign on the street, in the boardroom, and, yes, even in the yoga studio. For true balance to be restored in our bodies and our communities, this needs to change.

We need yoga practices that not only reunite us with our sensuality and body-based wisdom but also empower us to adapt our movements to complement our moods, energy levels, menstrual cycles, and stages of life. Because our bodies are microcosms of the earth herself — moving through cycles and made up of water, wood, fire, earth, and metal — we must find ways to get out of our minds and into the depths of our feeling bodies, daily. Doing so restores trust in our felt experience of being alive and dispels fears that we must control our bodies and hide their natural rhythms (with douches, tampons, diets, and even pills to stop menses altogether). When we start to feel and listen to our bodies daily through conscious movement, we stop running, controlling, and perfecting and learn to rest in all of who we are.

To sum up our discussion, the core qualities of women's yoga include yin yoga postures to cultivate receptivity, softness, patience, and letting go, as well

YIN AND YANG

The well-known yin/yang symbol from Taoism illustrates how the coessential, yet polarized, masculine (yang) and feminine (yin) energies intermingle and flow together to create a balanced whole. Ultimately, Taoists believe that everything in nature is infused with this dynamic interplay of yin and yang. Each man holds feminine, or yin, qualities, just as each woman holds masculine, or yang, qualities to different degrees. When we appropriately balance these two poles, we become integrated human beings.

Here are some key aspects of yin and yang to help you get to know the essential qualities of each of these better:

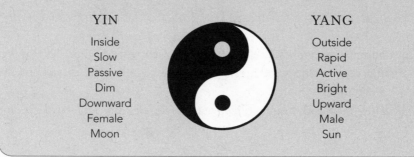

YIN	YANG
Inside	Outside
Slow	Rapid
Passive	Active
Dim	Bright
Downward	Upward
Female	Male
Moon	Sun

as the capacity to abide in loving presence with unpleasant, pleasant, and neutral sensations; yang (or flow) yoga postures to build the stamina, strength, perseverance, fluidity, and steady grace that come from moving in synchronization with the breath; a turning away from language and technical concepts to inhabit the right side of the brain; regular cycles of rest and activity that mirror the cycles of day/night, new moon/full moon, menstruation/ovulation, the four seasons, and so on; creative expression, intuitive movement, valuing the process over perfection, and devotion to the practice rather than rigid discipline. Please note that more yoga and meditation video instruction as well as a two-CD *Women's Yoga Kit* (with a yin and a yang practice) are available on my website, www.TheWayoftheHappyWoman.com.

YIN YOGA

Sometimes called the "quiet practice," yin yoga calms and quiets the mind, bringing you to a sense of inner peace that's helpful for seated meditation. It also soothes the nervous system and encourages energy flow and circulation through the joints and organs.

For times when you're feeling overstimulated, excessively extroverted, distraught, or burned out (an abundance of yang energy), yin yoga is a good antidote. This quiet, contemplative practice provides the space for true wisdom and healing to arise. It includes passive, floor-based postures (done with little or no muscular engagement), each of which you hold for one to five minutes. They usually target the lower body: the legs, hips, and lower back, or those regions closer to the spine and the vital organs in the core of the body. Yin postures teach us to value slowness, steadiness, stillness, and an attitude of total surrender and receptivity. These postures are perfect for when you're feeling run-down or sick or when you're menstruating, and, moreover, you don't need a yoga mat or any props to do them. One of my antidotes to jet lag is to do yin yoga on my hotel bed before I go to sleep at night. It always works wonders.

Yin postures might look sweet and soothing (which they are, ultimately), but newcomers to the practice will tell you that these poses can be quite challenging internally, since they do elicit strong physical and emotional sensations. In each posture you go to "the edge" — that gap between a pose being too easy and its being injurious — of what you can tolerate in order to stress a certain area of the body and to increase circulation and induce healing there. In yin yoga we stress the more yin tissues: our bones, ligaments, joints, and connective tissue.

Stemming from Taoist yoga, these postures also work like self-administered needleless acupuncture sessions and can be a potent form of self-healing. They place pressure on the energetic highways in the body called meridians — of which there are twelve main ones, each associated with one of six different yin/yang organ pairs. When we compress these meridians in still postures held for long periods (just as when a needle is placed on an acupuncture point), energy is activated or quieted along these unseen inner pathways, depending on what's needed to restore balance. Another benefit of practicing yin yoga is that while the postures are passive, the mind remains alert and focused.

BEGINNER'S TIP

When practicing yin yoga, start with holding each pose for one minute, then gradually work up to the more advanced holding time of five minutes. Also, you might find it easier to practice yin yoga after yang (flow) yoga, since your mind is more focused and your body more open, and you won't feel as restless.

For yin yoga to be effective, it's important to follow these three core principles, which my teacher Sarah Powers, one of the pioneers of yin yoga, outlines as:

1. *Come to your appropriate edge.* Enter a shape with sensitivity. You know that you've gone too far if your breath or body tenses up. If that happens, back up until you find ease again. When you tense up, your chi can't flow and you're being counterproductive; so only come to a point where you can stay relaxed.
2. *Become still and muscularly soft.* Give in to the hug of gravity. Let your muscles go. When you do this, chi can move from exterior to interior — away from your muscles and into your bones and joints.
3. *Hold each pose for one to five minutes.* Just as an acupuncturist doesn't put needles in and take them out right away, you need to stay in each position for a while — long enough to move chi effectively through your meridians.[2]

YANG (OR FLOW) YOGA

Sometimes the circumstances of our lives call for a quiet, more restorative practice, and we need to listen to this. However, for most of us, most of the time, we need both a yin and a yang practice. With too much yin we can become spacey and disconnected from our will. With too much yang we can become overly driven and desensitized to our inner callings. Therefore, it's best to couple yin yoga with yang, or flow, yoga.

I define flow yoga as dynamic, rhythmic movement aligned with the breath and embraced by mindfulness. This practice cultivates our inner fire and a lustrous and awake quality of body and mind. Held in short durations, yang postures strengthen and lengthen muscles. One flows in and out of poses, guided by the rhythm of the breath. Unlike yin yoga, which primarily bypasses the muscles to get to the deeper ligaments and joints, flow yoga requires muscular engagement and, in turn, stimulates blood flow and energy to our muscular bodies.

When we practice these two approaches over time, we enhance our intuition about what to practice when. For instance, sometimes I find it beneficial to do a yin practice in the morning and a hike in the afternoon. The next day I might do a yang practice or go to a dance class and do a yin practice in the evening before bed. On cold winter mornings, or when you're feeling less flexible, you can start with a warming flow practice and conclude it with long-held, quieting yin postures. The possibilities are endless and allow lots of opportunity to adapt your practices so they act as medicine for the different layers of your being — body, mind, emotions, and spirit.

SACRED BOOKENDS: INTENTION AND DEDICATION

While in our journey together we seek to marry the sacred with the mundane in each moment of each day, during your formal practice time it's imperative to consciously step away from habitual living and get crystal clear about your deepest intentions for practice. This precision brings great power to your practice time, even if you only have ten minutes.

Here's how:

- *Check in.* When you take a seat on your cushion or mat, first notice your inner landscape. Do this by checking in with each of the four layers of your being — body, mind, emotions, and spirit. I recommend doing this as often as possible, ideally at least three or four times a day. You can practice it when you wake up in the morning, before you sit down for lunch, before you go to sleep at night, or any time you're feeling disconnected from yourself. If you're new to this kind of self-investigation, start by checking in with your body. If you have more experience, add more layers — your mind, then your emotions. When you become more advanced you can include your spirit.
  1. *Body.* First bring your attention to your physical body. What position are you in? How does your body feel? Is she tired, energized, sore? Is a particular part calling for attention?
  2. *Mind.* This might be the easiest of the four to connect with since, for better or worse, we're so often lost in thought. Ask yourself, What are

my thoughts right now? What have I been thinking about for the past few hours?

3. *Emotions.* Here's where we have the least amount of awareness — and vocabulary. We live in a world that doesn't make space for our emotions. Come up with at least three adjectives that describe how you're feeling. Examples include bored, excited, confused, hopeless.

4. *Spirit.* This is the time when you check in with your intuition — that small, quiet voice inside that will grow bigger and louder when you turn to it frequently. Ask yourself, "What do I need to know right now?" Whatever answer arises — the first thing that comes up, either as an inner voice or just a flash of knowing — is your highest self, your spirit, speaking to you.

- *Set your intention.* This can be a personal intention for healing, balance, or clarity and ease with a challenge you're facing. I have found it really helpful to use the one taught to me by Sarah Powers: "I vow now to open to awareness for the benefit of all beings. I appreciate its immeasurable value. I feel it is possible for me in this moment, regardless of conditions and inclusive of all circumstances." This reminds me that the efforts I put into healing myself will also heal others — and that no matter what chaos or calamities may be whirling around me, true peace and healing are always possible.

- *Dedicate the merit.* To create a sacred seal at the end of your practice, remind yourself again of why these efforts are so important for you and for the world. A simple phrase from the Buddhist tradition that I like to use is "I dedicate the merit of my practice to the benefit of all beings."

As we move through our year together, we will experience these three aspects of practice with great intimacy, for we'll explore a different yin yoga, flow yoga, and meditation practice for each season. But before we dive into those, let's also take a look at the fundamental principles and practices of your outer world — primarily nutrition and sacred, seasonal eating and cooking.

REMEMBER

- Marry the sacred with the mundane by letting your outer world blossom from a rich inner life.
- Mindfulness is simply paying attention to what is. Participate in everything you see, feel, hear, taste, and smell every day. Be aware of your breath. Be aware of your thoughts too (but don't get lost in them).

- Inject periods of silence into your day, and consider going on a silent retreat.
- Check in with your intuition by asking, "What do you want me to do now?"
- When a strong emotion comes up, rather than pushing it away, see where you feel it in your body. Touch the qualities of these feelings with your awareness as they live and change inside you.
- Find ways to bring both receptive and dynamic activities into each day. Infuse your spiritual practice with rest, activity, and reflection to nurture and balance all parts of yourself.
- Practice checking in regularly with the four layers of your being: body, thoughts, emotions, and spirit.

Chapter 4

A WOMAN'S OUTER WORLD
Sacred Nutrition

Whenever I move into a new home, I always unpack the kitchen first. The kitchen is where life happens: families convene, heart-to-heart conversations happen, and we prepare and eat the very food that keeps us alive. When we consume wholesome foods, our bodies extract energy from the earth and transform it into the medicinal substance we need in order to think, move, regenerate cells, and much more. Both *what* and *how* we ingest inform how we look and feel, making food the most tangible, accessible, and ultimately pleasurable pathway to cultivating a rich outer world. Food gives us the sustenance we need to manifest our inner promptings and desires in our daily lives.

Whether it's through shopping for, eating, cooking, or reading and thinking about it, women come to life around food. Like us, it embodies fullness, diversity, healing powers, sensuality, and nurturance. However, many factors have eroded our healthy alliance with food. The rampant use of pesticides, overworking the land, water and air pollution, eating disorders, a cultural obsession with thinness, compulsive busyness, microwaves, and fast food all contribute to our disconnection from food, and, in turn, from our bodies and the earth herself. Through healing our relationship with food we restore balance and grateful reciprocity between ourselves and nature.

BARE CUPBOARDS

I need more than two hands to count the number of women around the world with whom I've had the good fortune of staying during my travels who *never* use their kitchens. Equipped with stacks of take-out menus, they leave their cupboards and refrigerators bare of anything fresh, vibrant, and colorful. They've forgotten the power of cutting one's own vegetables, brewing an herbal tea, or simply steaming a pot of rice. In these homes I unzip my totes and reveal my hidden loot: brown rice, mung beans, spices, a green powder blend, sea salt.

Many of these women come to me with complaints about their health: anxiety, irregular menstruation, acne, poor sleep, constipation, infertility. What I share with them is nothing new or profound. Rather, it's profoundly *simple*. I always start with noticing what a person is taking in — through their food, drink, environment, relationships, and thoughts. Getting involved with your food with *joy*, *reverence*, and *love* is crucial to building a life infused with happiness and health. I arrived at this understanding through my own initial disconnection from food, through trial and error, and through continued communion with food as a sacred entity.

Considering how poorly I ate when I was growing up, it's a miracle that I grew at all (it must have been those vitamins my grandmother slipped me whenever she came to visit!), much less came to adore vegetables, cooking, and anything and everything related to natural foods. I attribute the dramatic shift in my tastes to Ayurveda; regular cycles of cleansing and purification; and intuitive, conscious eating.

> ## TRY THIS
>
> In your journal, use the following questions to reflect on how you related to food as a child.
>
> 1. My favorite childhood foods were:
> 2. A typical family meal felt _____ and _____.
> 3. Three things we often talked about were:
> 4. The main lessons I learned about growing food, cooking it, and eating it when I was young were:
> 5. My two most positive childhood memories regarding food are:
> 6. My two most disturbing childhood memories regarding food are:
> 7. Three words that characterize my mother's relationship with food and cooking are:

AYURVEDA

I first learned about Ayurveda when I moved to Thailand. Ayurveda, the healing science of ancient India, means "the wisdom of life," for it gives us the tools to heal ourselves in the deepest sense and to discover, and live, our unique potential. It restores harmony within us and between us and our environment by balancing the *doshas* and the five elements of which they are composed — space, air, earth, fire, and water. These elements make up everything in the universe, including your body and the way your mind works (when you're agitated you have more fire, and when you have a cold you have more water). Clear signs of elemental harmony are that the body is clear of toxins, the mind rests at peace, emotions are calm and happy, organs function normally, and wastes are efficiently eliminated.

Since my own digestion was a mess from years of disordered eating, I gave it a try. First I took a *dosha* test to determine my unique constitution (you can take one online for free or, more accurately, with an Ayurvedic physician). We're all a combination of three *doshas* — *pitta*/fire, *vata*/air and space, and *kapha*/earth and water — in different degrees. Immediately, by making a few shifts, I experienced dramatic results. My appetite increased, and my digestion improved.

In addition to eating foods according to your constitution, at the heart of this approach to eating is choosing foods that are seasonal, local, and as close to their natural state as possible. This teaches you to eat for your life force by using food as your medicine. Eating local, seasonal foods tunes you in to the seasons and the dominant phytonutrients in nature, thus helping you to tune in to your needs even more. We cultivate those feelings we long to have more of in our lives: lightness, energy, clarity, and ease. Plus, when you buy local you support farmers and reduce your carbon footprint.

Here's a great example of the positive effects of eating a cleaner and more seasonal, local diet. A few years ago, Mike, a strong yogi with the physique of a football player, came to Thailand to attend my yoga teacher training. He had been serving in the military in Iraq, eating mostly convenient, processed foods, heavy on the meat. At one point in the course students partake in a weekend meditation retreat, in which they eat a very light, vegetarian diet so that they can spend more time in meditation without falling asleep.

Mike declared at the end of the course that his biggest realization had nothing to do with yoga or meditation but was about how much better, lighter, and more energetic he felt after eating more vegetables! Now, if he can do it, anyone can!

I'm not saying you should become a vegetarian for life, since I myself eat high-quality animal products when my body tells me she needs them. I *am* suggesting that you give it a try for a short period of time as an experiment, to notice how it makes you feel. On discovering just how good they feel afterward, many people, like Mike, decide to eat more fresh, vibrant foods.

TRY THIS

According to Ayurveda, an important precursor to good health is a healthy digestive fire. When your digestion's off, everything else will be too. Keeping your inner fire strong every day through simple rituals is one of the best preventative measures you can take for your health. Here are simple ways to do that, year-round:

1. *Drink ginger tea.* Ginger kindles the digestive fire. You can start your morning with a hot cup of ginger tea and sip it throughout the day, especially at mealtimes. Consider adding minced ginger root to your soups and stir-fries, and even chewing on a slice of ginger before your meals.

2. *Eat local, seasonal foods.* Familiarize yourself with the foods that grow in your area at different times of the year. Luckily, this is becoming easier now that more and more people are doing it — even President Obama! Eating this way aligns your body's rhythms to those of the outer world and strengthens your overall immunity and vibrancy. I'll give you detailed lists and recipes for how to do this in the coming chapters.

3. *Eat three meals a day.* Ayurveda recognizes 10:00 A.M. to 2:00 P.M. as the time when the sun's power, and the digestive force, is strongest, so make lunch your biggest meal of the day.

4. *Do a twelve-hour fast, every day.* Ayurveda, TCM, and many ancient healing traditions from around the world say the same thing: don't eat anything between dinner and breakfast. In fact, that's exactly why the latter is called what it is: you should be "breaking your fast" every morning. Go to sleep about three to four hours after dinner, refrain from late-night snacks, and go to bed around 10:00 P.M. When you've eaten three balanced meals during the day, most likely your body will feel satisfied and you won't need to snack as much. However, by fasting for twelve hours every night — between dinner and breakfast (7:00 P.M. to 7:00 A.M., for example) — you free your body from the burdens of meal-related digestion so it can conduct mental, emotional, and cellular cleansing in a more concentrated way as you sleep. This fast supports metabolism, prevents accumulation of toxins, normalizes weight, and, overall leaves you feeling clear and energized when you wake up in the morning — rather than with that icky bloated, groggy feeling.

5. *Follow the sun and the seasons.* Attune yourself to the rising and setting of the sun by going to sleep at 10:00 P.M. and waking up with or before the sun. Shift your diet according to the time of year. Favor warm and grounding foods such as soups and stews in the fall and winter and lighter and cooler foods such as fruits and salads in the spring and summer.

6. *Forget the ice cubes.* If you want to keep a fire burning, don't throw water on it! Cold, frozen, and leftover foods (older than twenty-four hours) create congestion. Favor warm (or at least room-temperature) drinks and foods, especially if you're sick or your digestion is sluggish to begin with. The only

exception to this is in the summertime when it's really hot outside, when there's nothing better than a cold drink.

MY APPROACH

Both Ayurvedic and Taoist perspectives influence all the recipes in this book. They favor local, seasonal foods to harmonize your body with the dominant environmental elements and to support the organ systems activated during those months (purifying foods in the spring to strengthen the liver and gall-bladder, cooling foods in the early summer to assist the heart and small intestine and in the late summer to assist the spleen and stomach, grounding foods in the autumn to soothe the large intestine and lungs, and warming foods in the winter to recharge the kidneys and bladder).

Also, all the recipes emphasize plenty of fresh vegetables, fruits, and grains. They are all vegetarian and dairy- and gluten-free (gluten is a protein found in starches such as wheat, barley, and rye, which many people are allergic to, the most extreme case being those with celiac disease) in order to accommodate the widest range of people possible. I have purposely omitted the popular vegan protein sources of unfermented soy products such as tofu and soy milk from these recipes, since they're hard to digest for most and can upset the estrogen balance in one's body if eaten in excess. If you eat meat, you are welcome to add some high-quality animal protein to the recipes if you'd like. If you experience fogginess, fatigue, bloating, gas, diarrhea, or constipation, you might be suffering from a food allergy, and the best thing to do is to go get tested and then to cut out one thing at a time (like dairy) for seven days and see how you feel. You will feel the best, though, if you adapt these recipes for your particular constitution, since eating is never one-size-fits-all.

THE HEALING ART OF COOKING

The next step in healing your relationship with food is befriending the art of cooking. What if you stopped viewing cooking as a chore and started thinking of it as a potent tool for transformation and connection? Preparing your own food is one the best ways to engage in self-healing and to connect with yourself and others. Just think of the classic book *Like Water for Chocolate* by Laura Esquivel. By preparing food with love and conscious intention, the cook transmits powerful emotions into the food, and then into the bodies and hearts of others.

TRY THIS

To inspire yourself to spend more time in your kitchen and to bolster healthier eating habits, you need to stock up on the right ingredients. I know it might seem overwhelming, so go at your own pace. Every woman has a different level of readiness. If you're just getting started, experiment with brown rice noodles for dinner instead of your usual pasta. If you naturally gravitate toward these things, try replacing white sugar entirely with the alternatives below. Don't feel like you need to do all or nothing here.

TO THROW OUT/COMPOST/RECYCLE

- artificial sweeteners (NutraSweet, Equal, Sweet'n Low, Splenda)
- white sugar (including products containing it — look at the ingredients in breakfast cereals, sodas, juices, yogurts, granola, "health" bars, etc.)
- white flour (including products containing it, such as white bread, pasta, baking mixes, pastries, cookies)
- partially hydrogenated or hydrogenated fats and oils (margarine, packaged baked goods, nonstick cooking sprays)
- canned foods laden with sugar, salt, and preservatives
- foods containing artificial coloring
- any food boasting an ingredients list a mile long, mostly of things you don't recognize

FOR YOUR PANTRY

(For simplicity's sake, please assume that every ingredient I list is organic.)

- extra virgin, cold-pressed olive oil in a dark glass bottle
- balsamic vinegar
- seaweeds (dulse, kelp, nori, kombu, and any others you like)
- course, unrefined sea salt
- grains such as quinoa, brown rice, rolled oats, millet, wild rice, and any others you like, stored in tightly sealed glass jars
- legumes such as lentils, garbanzo beans, mung beans, black beans, adzuki beans, and any others you like, stored in tightly sealed glass jars
- spices such as cinnamon, bay leaves, garlic powder, ground thyme, whole cumin, ground coriander, turmeric, salt-free curry powder, dried ginger, cloves, whole black peppercorns, paprika, mustard seeds, rosemary, sage, cayenne pepper, oregano, cardamom, stored in tightly sealed glass jars
- sun-dried tomatoes
- gomasio

- vegetable stock
- canned tomatoes and tomato paste
- olives
- sweeteners such as raw honey, agave nectar, maple syrup, stevia, and xylitol (more about these on page 151)
- cold-pressed coconut oil
- herbal teas such as ginger, chamomile, peppermint, Yogi DeTox, and rooibos
- raw apple cider vinegar
- brown rice protein powder
- carob powder
- brown rice pasta
- canned beans (no salt added) and jarred or canned tomato sauces for when you need to make a quick meal
- light, unsweetened coconut milk
- vanilla extract
- sesame oil
- dried, unsulfured and unsweetened fruits, including coconut
- energy bars (I like Lärabars and Organic Food Bars)
- brown rice cakes (unsalted)

FOR YOUR REFRIGERATOR

- tamari (wheat-free soy sauce) or Bragg's Liquid Aminos
- nuts and seeds (raw and unsalted), such as almonds, flaxseeds, pecans, walnuts, cashews, pine nuts, pumpkin seeds, sesame seeds, and sunflower seeds, kept in your freezer
- nut butters such as almond butter and tahini
- dates and raisins
- specialty foods such as green powder, spirulina, maca, and other superfoods (more about these on page 95)
- seasonal produce (shopping lists for each season coming in later chapters)
- unpasteurized miso
- organic eggs
- frozen fruits and vegetables for when you need to make a quick meal
- dark chocolate (70 to 80 percent cacao)
- unsweetened coconut water
- chia seeds (kept in your freezer)
- sprouted or gluten-free bread
- lemon juice, unpasteurized
- Dijon mustard

Have you ever been to a restaurant where the cook and wait staff seemed grumpy and impatient? How did you feel after eating your meal? Probably not very satisfied, and perhaps a little agitated yourself! Contrast that to sharing a meal with a friend in her home. Perhaps she prepared something simple, like lentil soup, homemade bread, and a green salad. But she's been chopping, stirring, and seasoning all afternoon while humming and listening to her favorite music, happily anticipating your arrival. Then, in the evening, you both savor the meal over a glass of red wine and candlelight. You share an intimate and scintillating conversation, and you leave feeling immensely satisfied. Energy is malleable. It can move through you, into your food, and into your body or the bodies of others. But before you cook for others, begin with cooking for yourself.

When we step into the kitchen and immerse ourselves in fresh ingredients, we also dive deeply into our sensuality. Chopping vegetables and pounding spices, we tune in to an ancient rhythm and start to align ourselves with the food that will soon become a part of us.

I know that we don't always have a lot of time to spend in the kitchen. There's a way to eat well and to have fun in the process with simplicity and flair, and that's exactly what I'll teach you how to do in the coming chapters. Each recipe I've selected is meant to bring you maximum nourishment without complicated instructions and ingredients. Each will ideally inspire you to come up with your own innovative ways of combining ingredients and becoming an artist in your kitchen. Make it an event! Turn on music, sing, chant, and invite your children to join in with you. They love to stir (and, of course, to lick the spoon and bowl afterward).

THIS IS NOT A DIET!

The food guidelines shared here are not in any way intended to add more guilt, self-hatred, and rigidity to your relationship with eating. They're here to reveal a pathway to making empowered decisions in your kitchen, grocery store, or restaurant that ultimately bring you more freedom, pleasure, and radiant health. Your participation, self-inquiry, and curiosity stand at the other end of my intention. I urge you to find the pleasure! See what works for you and see what doesn't. Your body's the ultimate authority. Just know that it's possible to restore a way of eating and being around food that's spontaneous, organic (double meaning intended), joyful, and easy. In fact, that's how it's *supposed* to be.

After many years of being incredibly restrictive with my food, I know all too well what it feels like to crave something and to ignore the craving. The result: I end up eating something I'm not in the mood for (but think I should eat), all in the name of trying to drone out that underlying need. I think if I ignore it, it will go away. Wrong! It's far better to eat something you're craving in moderation than to binge on it later or to eat something you don't really want. And if after reading this you're still afraid of giving in to intuitive wisdom (or even baffled about how to go about it) because you feel as if your body will betray you or that this kind of process has gotten you into trouble before, don't worry. Staying present to yourself and open to rediscovering yourself during this journey will bring you to a place of trusting, revering, and listening to your body's wisdom.

CONSCIOUS EATING

One vital way to tap into intuitive eating is to simply slow down when you eat. We can all relate to scarfing down a burrito in the car during rush-hour traffic or gobbling down a snack bar while running to catch the train. Nowadays, it is easy to neglect the sacredness of our food. But the quality of foods that you eat, and the attention that you give to the act of eating, deeply affects your health and consciousness. When you take time to enjoy your food, you become attuned to what your body wants and when she's had enough. Plus, you'll notice that you end up eating *less* and enjoying what you're eating *more* when you slow down and notice.

To support healthy digestion and optimal enjoyment, choose a relaxing and comfortable eating venue — ideally without TV, books, magazines, or other distractions. When I visit a restaurant, sometimes that means asking for a table farther away from the heavily trafficked entrance. At home it means setting a place at the table, turning away from the computer, or resisting reading a magazine. Less-than-optimal dining scenarios are unavoidable facts of life, and, for most of us, it is a challenge to make time for a conscious eating practice at every meal! Increase your chances of success by choosing at least one meal a day when you can fully practice and be present with your food. Then for the other meals, incorporate what you can from the list below.

TEN STEPS TO CONSCIOUS EATING

1. *Hydrate.* Always keep a glass of water nearby you as you're working, or carry a water bottle with you wherever you go. Aim to drink liquids between twenty minutes and one hour before eating. Drinking liquids during meals dilutes digestive enzymes and the stomach's hydrochloric acid, thus

impairing digestion. If you must have a beverage with a meal, drink small amounts of warm water (with lemon is nice) or an herbal tea such ginger or peppermint (herbs that aid digestion). Avoid cold drinks, unless it's really hot outside, since these can dampen your digestive fire.

2. *Breathe deeply.* Before you eat, do several rounds of diaphragmatic breathing (especially if you're feeling emotional or stressed). This relaxes the nervous system and enhances blood flow to the digestive organs. It also helps you tune in to your body so that you eat only what your body needs.

3. *Extend gratitude.* Recite a blessing of gratitude for the food, the earth, and everyone involved in growing, preparing, and bringing the food to you. Sentiments of gratitude alone can boost the immune system!

4. *Engage the senses.* Take time to look at the food and appreciate its shapes, colors, and textures. Smell your food, and enjoy its aromas.

5. *Savor the first bite.* Let your first bite rest in your mouth, and see if you can detect what flavors are present.

6. *Chew well.* Chew slowly and thoroughly. Notice the impulse to swallow prematurely, and resist it. Try chewing your food as many as thirty times, to the point where it is liquefied. The more thoroughly you chew, the better your digestion will be.

7. *Slow down.* Take breaks to stop chewing and breathe. This calms your nervous system and encourages optimal digestion. In addition, by slowing down you can tune in to when you are full and, in this way, avoid overeating and overtaxing your digestive system. It is best to finish eating when you still feel slightly hungry, or when your stomach feels three-quarters full. There's no need to overindulge. You can always eat again later if you get hungry!

8. *Observe.* Turn your awareness inside your body — to your mouth and your belly — to be as present to the sensations of eating as possible. Notice what images, feelings, and inspirations arise for you as you eat. Whenever you find your mind wandering, bring it back to what you are doing: lifting the fork, chewing, swallowing, and putting the fork down.

9. *Complete the practice.* Take a few moments before getting up from your meal. Take a few deep breaths and/or once again extend gratitude to the food and the earth and beings who provided it.

10. *Notice the effects.* Be sure to notice how you digest your meals and whether

this practice has any positive effects on your body, your mind, or life in general.

Start putting some of these fundamentals into action. We'll return to them again and again as we step into the kitchen each season of the year. Now that we have laid the foundation for our journey, it's time to get clear about your vision and intentions so that you get the most out of this coming year.

REMEMBER

- Get involved with your food! Shop for it, chop it, smell it, cook it, eat it with joy and gusto.
- Cook for yourself with love. Then cook for others with love.
- Eat seasonally and locally. Emphasize lots of fruits, veggies, and whole grains.
- Practice listening to what your body wants to eat. When you pause and ask her what she wants, are you willing to listen?
- While eating, slow down, chew, and savor the experience.
- Stock your kitchen with the wholesome ingredients and supplies that you need to support your journey.
- Choose a relaxing and comfortable eating venue.

Chapter 5

PREReparing *for the* WAY

We're almost ready to get started. But before we really dig in, first let's make sure that we have two final bricks of our foundation in place: a sacred space into which you can retreat and recharge when you need to and some goals and intentions to steer you and keep you on the course of your heart's deepest desires. With these in place, you will be well on your way to the best year of your life.

CREATE A SACRED SPACE

For a practice to really take root in your life, it needs a container, or a sacred space. As Virginia Woolf so aptly wrote, every woman needs a room of her own.

Something I loved about my years of living and traveling in Asia was the ubiquitousness of sacred spaces: the spirit house that stood guard in the garden of my Thai home and the small offering tray of banana leaves, flowers, and incense that I nearly tripped over as I meandered through Balinese rice paddies. Now I have an altar covered with pictures of my teachers, as well as stones, shells, and feathers from all over the world (you can see a video tour of my altar on my website). Surrounded by these things, I'm reminded of what matters to me and of the kind of person I aspire to be. I see the sacredness, and the beauty of my own being, reflected back to me.

I know women who make little nooks for themselves in their closets or guest bedrooms. Some erect a tipi in the yard. If you don't already have such a space, set aside a room, or a corner of your room, that is yours and yours alone. Throughout our yearlong journey together you will need to return to your sacred space daily — for your yoga and meditation practices, as well as for journaling, being creative, praying, or simply resting and being alone. You'll know that whenever you sit, lie, or stand in this space, you'll be able to drop into a serene, contemplative state — free of work, spouses, and children. It's a place *just for you*. It's a place to connect with your rich inner world.

Monique, in California, is the mother of three children, all under five. A stay-at-home mom, she can't even go to the bathroom alone, much less have a whole room to herself. When I first met her, she was about to topple over from exhaustion. Full of excuses and anger, she insisted that there was absolutely no way she could create a sacred space for herself. "There's no such thing!" she insisted. I asked her to describe the layout of her bedroom. Then I suggested that she take out a decorative armchair in the corner and put up a folding screen to form a small, semicircle around that corner instead. The enclosure inside that screen would be her sacred space. She could put her meditation cushion in there, a blanket, and anything else she wanted. "Yes, yes, I can do that!" she responded with sudden enthusiasm. When she needed a time-out — when her children were napping or when her husband was home and she could hand them off to him for ten minutes — she now had a place to go. It's possible, even if it doesn't seem so at first, for every woman to create a sacred space.

YOUR ABSOLUTE YES AND ABSOLUTE NO LISTS

Now that your space is set up (or spruced up), take out your journal, and let's get clear on what you most desire to be, see, and do — specifically in the year ahead. By clearly acknowledging and naming the things that give you strength and inspiration — as well as those things that diminish your light — you're taking an empowered step toward living as your highest, most divine self amid the nitty-gritty of your daily life.

Start by making an Absolute Yes List, an exercise I learned from life coach and author Cheryl Richardson. Brainstorm all the things that make you a stronger, better person and that you absolutely can't live without. Eventually you will pare it down to around ten to twenty things. For example, on my list I have:

1. Sleep at least eight hours a night.
2. Take a candlelit bath a few times a week.
3. Do yoga six days a week, even if it's just for ten minutes.
4. Go for walks outside at least a few times a week.
5. Spend my mornings in silence.
6. Meditate a minimum of ten minutes a day.
7. Eat simple, wholesome foods that agree with me.

8. Get a pedicure every month and a massage every other week.
9. Dance at least once a week.
10. Write in my journal every day, including some thoughts on what I'm grateful for. Ideally three pages, but sometimes just a few words or a haiku if I don't have time.
11. Go on at least one meditation retreat and one beach vacation a year.
12. Meet up with friends at least a couple of times a week.
13. Visit the farmers' market on Saturday mornings.
14. Take a rest day after traveling before jumping back into things.
15. Totally unplug one day a week.

Whenever you start to get burned out or are preparing for a challenging situation (such as visiting your family over the holidays or meeting a big work deadline), refer back to your list. Make sure you're incorporating as much as you can from your Yes List.

It's also helpful to make an Absolute No List. As women we often want to please and serve everyone else so much that it's hard for us to say no. Natural helpers, sometimes we take on more than is healthy for us. When we do say no, we feel we need to follow it up with lengthy reasons and justifications. I advocate that when someone asks you to do something that doesn't feel like an absolute yes in your belly, just say no. That's it. No excuses. No justifications. No apologies. Simply say, "I can't do that." Speaking from personal experience, you will feel uncomfortable! You'll want to explain, to try to make the other person like you — but resist this impulse. Saying no to everything that's not an absolute yes gives you back your power. Each time you stomach through (I use that term because we often do things with a knot in the belly) something that you don't really want to do, you're hurting yourself.

Just as you did above with your Absolute Yes List, jot down around ten to twelve things that you know weaken, irritate, and lead you away from who you truly are. Here are some things on my Absolute No List:

1. No checking email first thing in the morning or last thing at night.
2. No laptop in bed unless I'm watching a movie.
3. No working on Sundays.
4. No strenuous activity or work on the first day of my moon time.
5. No red-eye flights.
6. No letting things slide and not speaking up for what I want or need.

7. No call waiting. Disable the function on my phone so that conversations can't be interrupted.
8. No competing with or comparing myself to others.
9. No checking email more than a few times a day or zoning out on the Internet for more than thirty minutes.
10. No excuses for not letting my body move or get outside every day, unless I'm sick.
11. No eating when I'm angry, upset, or having a stressful conversation.

You can keep your Yes and No Lists, as well as your journal, in your sacred space throughout the year so that they're always there to support you. You don't need to live each point on the list each day, but they're anchors for you to come back to. They remind you of what you need to feel your best and serve as the breadcrumb trail back to your happiness. Remember, feeling good is *not* arbitrary; it's a practice and a responsibility! We're almost ready to move on, but first I want to share one important preliminary exercise to help you bring out your inner world and to focus the coming year on what you truly want.

IT TAKES THIRTY DAYS

It takes thirty days to form a new habit. (And if you're trying to *let go* of an old habit, it works the same way — you just need to replace that old habit with a new, healthy one.) The first step is deciding to do it. Commit to it. For example, if you want to start meditating for ten minutes every day when you wake up, write that down in your journal, and then add accountability by telling a friend about it or posting it on our Facebook forum (www.facebook.com/WayofHappy Woman). Then, no matter what outer or inner storms come your way, do it every day, sitting at the same time, in the same place, for thirty days. No excuses! The more consistent you are, the easier it will be for the habit to stick.

I've worked with women who have done yoga, walked, cut out sugar, quit smoking, or omitted red meat for thirty days straight. After that, it was much easier for them to keep up their new, healthier habits. If you're trying to cut down on your coffee intake, before the thirty days start to replace your regular coffee with decaf. Make sure you have supplies on hand to support you, not sabotage you. Mark your calendar for the first and last of these thirty days so you don't stop short of your goal, and then go for it. We will work on this together as we go, for in the final chapter of each season, you'll have a chance to decide on one habit to focus on cultivating each month.

TRUST YOUR EXPERIENCE

Feminine wisdom ripens through your bodily experience. This type of knowing, however, isn't very valued in the world today. But I encourage it. As a woman, you need to learn to trust yourself and your body. Our culture adores scientific proof — concepts that can be tested. Your bodily wisdom is different. It's knowing in your bones that something is so, because you're breathing it and know it for yourself. Dedicated practice changes you. It shows you what's true from deep inside you. It makes your own inner wisdom the supreme authority. And *that's* why practice is so powerful and not something you can skimp on.

Yes, you can read this book, and the concepts I share may elicit more richness in your life, but it's in day-to-day embodied practice (rather than just the intellectual act of reading) that you transform and ripen at a much deeper level. Everything I share here comes out of my own felt experience and from what has benefited me. That's the only place from which I can truly absorb my insights, and it's the only place from which I can then teach and write about them. I empower you to trust your *own* experience. This is the only way that you can move from your head to your heart. *Live* these things in *your* body. Stop expecting someone else to heal you, save you, or create your perfect life. Now's the time to become the healer, artist, and sage that you, as a woman, were born to be.

TRY THIS

Your girlfriends will be important allies on the journey ahead. Right now make a list of three or four women in your life whom you know you can call and share your deepest truths with. These are your go-to women to help you through rough patches, reflect back to you what you need to see, and celebrate your victories with you. Now, from this list, talk to one girlfriend on the phone or invite her out to tea or for a walk. The best scenario would be the two of you reading this book together, but if she's not on board with that, you can still make this work. Ask each other the following questions. Be sure to give each other enough time to answer thoroughly. Once you've finished, talk about what you learned from each other and what you're inspired to do with these findings.

1. What are the biggest sources of stress in your life right now?
2. How do they affect you?
3. What are the biggest sources of joy and calm in your life right now?
4. What one change could you make to your daily life that would create more joy and less stress?
5. How can I support you with this?
6. What other means of support do you have? (Consider other close friends, therapists, coaches, mentors, yoga teachers, acupuncturists, etc.)

THE YEAR AHEAD

Now it's time to get out your journal to clarify your intentions and vision for the coming year. Do set aside the time to do this, since you'll return to these again and again over the coming months to remind yourself why you're doing this and what really matters. We all come to low points when we doubt ourselves and want to quit. Writing down your goals and dreams will help you to get through those times. Countless studies have shown that those who take the time to map out their goals have higher success rates than those who don't. I want you to succeed, and I know you want to too!

1. The three things am I most longing to see, be, do, or experience in the year ahead are:
2. My top three spiritual goals for the next year are:
3. My top three professional goals for the next year are:
4. My top three personal/family/community goals for the next year are:
5. My top three health (physical, mental, and emotional) goals for the next year are:
6. The one main change that I absolutely would like to bring about in my everyday life this year is:
7. The one experience I most want to have this year is:
8. My three main fears about this journey are:
9. The thing about myself that I most want to learn to love and accept this year is _____, and the main thing that I think might hold me back from doing this is _____.
10. If I were to guess, my biggest obstacle to sticking with this journey will be _____. Some ideas that I have about how to overcome that when I face it are _____ and _____.
11. Some ways that I can use the power of friendship and community to support me through this are to _____ and _____.
12. To be totally honest, my biggest, boldest, and most outlandish desire for the year ahead that I'm almost afraid to even admit to myself is _____.
13. I rank my current priorities as follows: [Put a number to the left of each of the categories below. Feel free to tweak them to make them more relevant if needed. Then, on the right, number the categories *as you'd like them to be prioritized by the end of the year.*]

    ___ friends ___
    ___ finances ___
    ___ romance ___
    ___ health ___

__ spirituality   __
__ personal growth   __
__ career   __
__ family   __
__ community   __
__ fun/play/pleasure __

14. The main things that bring me joy and really make my soul sing (and that I vow to experience more of this year) include _____, _____, _____, and, most of all, _____.

15. One year from now, I'd love to read back over these words and feel _____, _____, and _____. I'd like to look _____ and _____ and be surrounded by _____ and _____.

Now close your eyes and see yourself as you would most like to be, one year from now. See the expression on your face, the light in your eyes, and the glow of your skin. What are you wearing, and how does it feel on your skin? What are you feeling? Take a few minutes to fully inhale, breathing in those emotions, feeling them deeply. Look around you — where are you? What are the colors, shapes, sounds, textures, and scents? Who is there with you? See and feel it all as fully as you can. Immerse yourself in this world for five minutes, drinking in all the details.

Once you open your eyes, make a visual representation of what you saw. Cut out pictures from a magazine, arrange them on a piece of poster board, and paste your own face on the bodies. If you're an artist, you can draw or paint your scene. Frame this or post it somewhere so that when you feel like throwing in the towel, you can remember what it's all about. You're on the path to embodying your highest, brightest, happiest self.

Now take a deep breath and tell me,

TRY THIS

If you notice that your inner critic starts acting up when you dream big, write down all the messages it's giving you. It will start to lose its power once you can see how ridiculous it is. Here are some examples of what your inner critic might say: "Are you crazy? There's no way you could ever do that!" "You'll never have enough money for that." "Yeah, right, keep dreaming." "You're going to stay exactly as you are and where you are."

Really let loose; write it all down. Then, once you feel complete, like a little girl having a temper tantrum, demolish that paper. Crumple it in your hands. Shred it. Throw it. Stomp on it. Burn it or flush it down the toilet and tell it what you really think of it! I know it sounds silly, but it's vital to involve your body, especially your voice, whenever your inner critic rears its ugly little head.

are you ready? Thank you for your patience as I laid out the basics for you. You're welcome to now jump ahead to the season that you're currently in and get started. If that season happens to be springtime, it's time to be reborn.... Here we go!

REMEMBER

- Set up a room, or some space of your own, and fill it with inspiring objects that remind you of all that is good, true, and beautiful about you and life.
- Make your Absolute Yes and Absolute No Lists. Keep them nearby. Turn to them when you feel like you're getting off track.
- Dream big! Get clear about what you want for yourself this year and then visualize it, feel it, live it.
- Acknowledge your inner critic when it appears. Give it voice by writing down what it's saying. Start realizing that this is not the voice of your spirit, so you don't need to give your power away to it.

PART 2

SPRING

Element: WOOD

Color: GREEN

Organs: LIVER AND GALLBLADDER

Heart qualities: ANGER AND LOVING-KINDNESS

Life cycle: CHILDHOOD

Creative cycle: BIRTH AND CREATION

Menstrual cycle: THE WEEK AFTER MENSTRUATION

Moon cycle: WAXING MOON

Actions: CREATIVE ACTION, DEVELOPMENT,
GROWTH, AND PLANNING

Focus: ACT ON YOUR DEEPEST VISION FOR RENEWAL,
REAWAKENING, AND REBIRTH.

Chapter 6

COMING *into* BEING

Every woman, whether or not she realizes it, is a creative genius. Within her lives the capacity to bring forth new life and to regenerate during each moon cycle and each spring. Life, and our vitality, bursts forth in the springtime. This season calls your innate creativity to awaken and make itself known, just as a seedling pushes through the thawing soil past roots and rocks toward the light. Now your visions and deep dreaming from the winter come into being. We begin our journey in the spring because it heralds your initiation and rebirth into a whole new you.

Officially arriving on March 21 with the spring equinox in the northern hemisphere (September 21 in the southern hemisphere), the spring exhales the intoxicating fragrance of radical possibility. Who do you want to be now? How do you want to live? What's ready to come to life inside you? We can always begin again. Green leaves emerging from barren branches, the first twitter of songbirds, and crocuses poking their way through melting snow: all symbolize your triumphant life force and spirit.

After the latency and visioning of winter's respite, we emerge in the spring-time with renewed energy. Fertile and full, like a newly blossomed lilac bush, our lives can have color, flair, and beauty. It's up to us to harness that energy. The potential's there for you, and the more you engage with it, the more you activate it. Through communal ritual and celebration, religions around the world recognize the magic of the springtime. Easter symbolizes resurrection from death and the immortality of spirit. Originally a pagan celebration of re-newal and rebirth, this holiday honored the Saxon goddess Eostre (also known as Ostara), who symbolizes springtime and fertility.

In the Jewish tradition, at Passover we praise the triumph of life over death, and we are asked to first taste the bitterness of any experience so that we may later appreciate its sweetness. Many Asian cultures celebrate their new year in the springtime. In Thailand you find Songkran, the infamous water festival that symbolizes the washing away of the previous year's baggage (and has become an opportunity for mammoth water fights in the streets!). Later in the season, around May 1, falls Beltane (also called May Day). Originally a Celtic festival of fire, praising the fertility of all things, Beltane is the traditional time for celebrations, marriage in particular, as well as a time for planting and caring for crops. All point back to spring's irresistible invitation to begin again.

Harness the power of this season as it supports you in the taking up of new, life-affirming habits: join a gym, commit to a regular meditation or yoga practice, or cut out white sugar from your diet. Now's the time to bring forth, through dedicated, focused action, all your heart's desires. Dare to dream big. Delve into your heart and bypass your mind. You'll know you're doing that when you start to feel excited, passionate, in love with your vision for your life. A flower doesn't stop herself from blossoming because she fears that she'll be too beautiful, colorful, or fragrant!

SPRING CLEANSING FOR YOUR HOME

In traditional Ayurveda, when a man and a woman want to become pregnant, they begin by cutting toxins out of their diets and stocking up on fertility-enhancing tonics. To give birth to new expressions of yourself, you need to do the same thing every spring. One of the easiest and most practical places to start clearing things out is your home.

Spring's the time to take charge of your life, and that begins with your living environment. Yes, it takes time and discipline, but there are no excuses here. Block off an hour, a day, or a weekend, and do it. Get help from your children, or hire a college student. Take it one step at a time, and remember that the first steps are the hardest. Once you take those, you'll have more momentum to carry you through. Be willing to be a bit uncomfortable, trust the process, and get started!

DECLUTTERING

The more clutter you have — in your home, car, or purse, or on your computer hard drive — the more your energy gets dissipated and called to the nonessentials. How much time do you spend looking for files (hard and soft) because you don't have a clear system in place? Here are some questions to ask as you go through your home, room by room, with the intention of simplifying and making space for new opportunities:

1. Does this lift my energy when I think about or look at it?
2. Is it genuinely useful? Did I use it last year?
3. Does it reflect who I want to be this year?
4. Does it make me feel powerful, beautiful, and confident? (This question works especially well when you get to your underwear drawer. Not sexy? Treat yourself to things that are!)

If you have a hard time letting go of objects with sentimental value, make three piles — one for things you'll keep, one for things you'll give away, and one for things you're not sure about. Then put the unsure pile in a box in the garage, basement, or attic. If you find that you don't open it in the next six to twelve months, see if you're ready to let the items go.

Even if you're not ready for the big sweep, at the very least open the windows, get a new houseplant, and burn incense or sage to purify the environment. Play upbeat music. Diffuse essential oils of tangerine and peppermint. Invite new life and energy into your home. You'll feel much lighter and freer at the end of your hard work!

I have a friend whose mother would move everyone's beds to invite in new perspectives at the start of each spring. My friend, who was a little girl at the time, always looked forward to the day she came home from school to find the new configuration, and she now does the same with her own daughter every year. What unique ways can you find to honor the turning of the season in your home environment?

SPRING CLEANSING FOR YOUR LIFE

As the days slowly become longer and brighter, they're beckoning *all* of you to awaken. This can feel difficult at first, since your body and emotions may have gotten comfortable with winter's more lethargic rhythm. Many of us have put on extra pounds during the past few months, a natural response to winter's chilly darkness. These extra pounds help to insulate and anchor us. In addition to weight gain, we might also be coping with some extra mucus (one way that your body releases toxins) due to spring allergies or with dull, depressed energy. It's time to enliven your body and your heart through a deep cleanse.

Bethany, a coaching client in Germany, felt stuck. Wife, business owner, and mother of three young children, she was completely exhausted and overwhelmed. Reliant on coffee to get her through her days, she had so many creative ideas brewing — a book, a DVD, a new boutique to open — yet she had no plan and didn't know where to even start looking for the time or energy to focus on these endeavors. She clearly had a spring imbalance. I suggested resting and taking time off, contemplating her unique dreams (regardless of the roles she played for others), and then being diligent in carving out time and space daily to birth these latent aspects of herself.

Here's the four-step plan Bethany used to bring the energy of rebirth back into her creative life:

1. Get childcare for one full day, from 9:00 A.M. to 5:00 P.M., and go on an artist date. Spend time in nature, browsing a favorite bookstore, going to a matinee solo. Get a massage or a pedicure. Do whatever makes you best come *alive*.

2. Find thirty minutes a day, six days a week, to inwardly reconnect. Maybe that means setting your alarm thirty minutes before the children wake up, or blocking off time when they're napping or before you go to sleep. Use the same time each day to build on the power of continuity. Divide your thirty minutes: fifteen minutes in meditation (using the Mindfulness Meditation, page 44) and then fifteen minutes writing in your journal. Write about what you dream of, what you desire most, what really matters to you.

3. Each day, take one step toward bringing your dreams to fruition. If the first dream you want to manifest is to open a boutique, scour real estate online to get price estimates and weigh the pros and cons of different neighborhoods. Do market research on similar stores and how yours would stand apart.

4. At the end of each day, write down everything that you did well and all the forward movement you made. The energy of wood, most dominant in the springtime, likes to root down and get grounded (through your self-care and introspection) while expanding and moving upward, like a tree. Celebrate growth, no matter how small it may seem!

One year later Bethany had opened her own children's clothing store and was starting to write a children's book. She did this through harnessing the momentum of spring: tapping into her desires and using the discipline that sprang from her dedication to create the plan needed to implement her dreams. She didn't get bogged down or overwhelmed. She simplified her vision and took clear, decisive steps to realize it.

THE WOOD ELEMENT

In Taoism and its sub-branch Traditional Chinese Medicine, the wood element is most dominant in the spring. Wood grows from the watery soil of wintertime.

From that incubation, it grows deep roots into the earth and surges forth into the light of the world to grow and expand. As the wind blows and the weather shifts, the tree stays stable and flexible, continually adapting to its environment to survive and thrive. It evolves through resilience.

Is there a tree in your yard or neighborhood that inspires you? Spend time near that tree. Sense its years and years of growth and stamina. Feel those same qualities in yourself. How can you have more faith in them? How can you bring them to the forefront? Tell the tree your dreams. Tell it how you need to be supported to grow. Ask it how it stays so rooted during turbulent times. You may be surprised to hear it talk back to you!

ONE-DAY SPRING RETREAT

To synthesize all the practices for this season, do a one-day spring retreat. If you live with your family, do this on a day when everyone's out of the house, or find a B and B or a country cabin where you can have one full day alone. Make sure you have all the supplies you need before you get started, and don't forget to unplug! Turn off your phone. Power down your computer. Return to distraction-free simplicity, and plan to spend the day in solitude and silence.

The earth's circadian rhythm shifts in the springtime with earlier sunrises and later sunsets, and the sleep/wake rhythm in your body shifts too. As the days grow longer, you need less sleep.

- Wake up between 5:00 and 7:00 A.M. Sleeping in will only make you feel lethargic and mentally dull. It's much better to go to sleep early (your liver, the organ most activated into detox mode this season, goes through a cycle of detoxification each night between 1:00 A.M. and 3:00 A.M. when you're sleeping). Take phlegm-conquering measures such as scraping your tongue and using the neti pot. Mucus is a sign that your body is trying to unload toxins this season.

- Drink a glass of warm lemon water on waking, followed by dandelion tea or Yogi DeTox tea. All these drinks stimulate cleansing of the liver. No coffee or black tea today. If you're hungry when you wake up, stir one tablespoon of psyllium seed husks into

SPRING RETREAT

a glass of water and drink immediately, followed by another tall glass of water. This helps to make you feel full while acting as a broom in your gastrointestinal track.

- Do the spring flow yoga sequence (page 113) or take a brisk walk, jog, swim, or bike ride. Make sure that you break a sweat, which will help with detoxifying.

- Do some skin brushing (page 83), give yourself a massage with sunflower oil (page 190), and take a hot, then cold, shower to boost lymphatic detox.

- Make the Spring Green Smoothie for breakfast (recipe on page 94).

- Choose a comfortable place to write in your journal for thirty minutes. Use some of the journaling topics discussed on pages 131–32, or write three or more pages about whatever feels true for you today.

- Sit outside near a tree or look at one out the window. Spend about five minutes in Mindfulness Meditation (page 44) and another five to ten minutes in Loving-Kindness Meditation (page 127).

- Make yourself some ginger tea (recipe on page 260) and read an inspiring book about health, nutrition, and cleansing. Prepare steamed kale and brown rice.

- Do any household chores that you need to do with sacred attention and mindfulness for one or two hours. Drink another tall glass of water with lemon.

- Sit for ten minutes in Mindfulness Meditation. Drink a tall glass of water with lemon.

- Do the spring yin yoga sequence for one hour (page 108).

- Prepare a dinner of either another Spring Green Smoothie (the most cleansing option) or steamed quinoa and asparagus with some lemon juice.

- Go for a slow, leisurely walk after dinner for thirty minutes. Drink a tall glass of water with lemon.

- Take a hot detoxifying salt bath (1 cup sea salt, 2 cups baking soda, 1 cup Epsom salts). Drink a tall glass of water with lemon afterward.

- Lights out at 10:00 P.M. Sweet dreams!

THE SKINNY ON YOUR SKIN

Your largest eliminative organ, your skin completes one quarter of your body's detoxification every day. It's the last organ to receive nutrients from your food and the first to show signs of imbalance and deficiency (hint: if you want to have beautiful skin, eat well, sleep well, and drink lots of water!). Another way to care for your skin daily is through skin brushing.

Scandinavians, Turks, and Russians have been in on this healing ritual for centuries. Not only does it slough off dead cells to make skin silky soft, but dry brushing also helps to remove cellulite; boost digestion, circulation, and detoxification; cleanse the lymphatic system; stimulate hormonal secretions; and strengthen the immune system.

Get a soft natural brush with a long handle so that you can reach all areas of your body. When I travel I bring a pair of exfoliation gloves with me. Get naked and brush your body — while it's still dry — right before bathing. Use long, sweeping strokes from the bottom of your feet up toward your torso, then from your hands up to your shoulders, and around your torso up to your heart. Stroke toward your heart to stimulate flow in the direction in which your veins travel.

Don't use too much pressure, especially where your skin's more sensitive. Brush lightly around your breasts. Be sure to reach the areas where lots of glands live — in your groin, armpits, and around your neck. Make circular strokes around your belly. Massage in oil now (see page 190). Take a shower, and finish with a one-minute blast of cold water (or, if you're feeling brave, do three thirty-second intervals of hot and cold blasts to stimulate circulation).

Be patient. It may take up to thirty days for you to start seeing and experiencing the wonderful changes that this practice, along with the others shared here, will bring as your liver clears up and its energy, or chi (more about this in the next two chapters), starts to move more freely and harmoniously through your body.

SPRING MOON TIME PRACTICES

One common sign that your liver chi has become stagnant is PMS, and PMS is a warning bell from your soul. Tory, a client of mine in California, suffered from such intense menstrual cramps each month that they made her nauseated. She also experienced terrible mood swings. She had tried everything: the Pill, homeopathy, acupuncture. I asked her, "Are you happy?" The line was silent for a few moments. "No, I'm not," she admitted. For the next hour we looked at the things in her life that weren't working for her: She hated her job but felt uninspired to find a new one, she suspected her boyfriend was cheating on her, and she often felt so depressed at the end of the day that she settled for a slice of pizza or a bag of chips for dinner.

Each month her body and emotions were desperately trying to catch her attention. She needed to make serious changes: finding an outlet for her creativity and passion, reclaiming her voice and power by standing up to her boyfriend, and eating foods that supported — rather than taxed — her body, her liver in particular. She had a lot of work to do but was desperate to feel good again. Over the next six months things gradually got better and better for her. She found a new job at an ad agency that let her put some of her creativity to use, she asked her boyfriend to move out and was dating again, and she had done a liver detox.

In your life, when PMS strikes, find the answers within for how to change and emerge renewed and refreshed after your menses. If you ignore the warning bells of PMS, you're setting yourself up for a more turbulent ride through menopause — since this rite of passage calls women to wake up to all the ways they've been ignoring their inner wisdom and to go after what they really want. Now let's step into the kitchen to take a closer look at how to cleanse our bodies through wholesome foods to invite more clarity, energy, and vitality this spring.

REMEMBER

- Revisit your reflections from chapter 5. Renew your commitment to them, or change them, if need be. During this expansive spring season, what do you want to see, be, or do over the next three months?
- Clean out your closets. Organize your office. Declutter your purse. Spring cleanse your surroundings to make more room for new people, projects, and opportunities.
- Break out of winter stagnation. Get up early. Hit the gym, get on your yoga mat, sweat, or do whatever you need to do to get moving. Be persistent!

Chapter 7

IN *the* KITCHEN
Clean and Green

Spring means green, and green symbolizes healing and renewal. The lime-colored buds on trees and the reemergence of grass from the brown earth bring a fresh, alive energy to the world. I have a friend who felt very run-down, on the verge of extreme burnout. Going around and around on the proverbial hamster wheel of busyness, he was stuck in a pattern of overworking, often leaving the house at 7:00 A.M. and not returning home until 9:00 or 10:00 at night — six days a week! Devoid of any time or energy to spend with his family, much less to nurture himself, he went to see a local healer who advised him to spend a minimum of one hour a week somewhere green. She told him to sit there and drink in the color through all his senses — to let it seep in through his eyes, to touch it, smell it. This simple act of connecting with the color of Mother Nature's vitality helped him to renew and rebalance. Similarly, a Celtic tradition on Beltane calls for everyone to wash her or his face in the morning dew at sunrise, to make love outdoors, and, for menstruating women, to roll around naked in the dewy grass. All these customs coax you to absorb spring's green fertility and vitality.

One essential way to invite more green into your life this season is to eat more green foods. Look around you — they're everywhere in the springtime! Especially if you meander through any farmers' market, you'll notice that the local foods at this time of the year include sprouts, spinach, dandelion greens, arugula, and asparagus. Yes, it's simple. But the effects go deep. Many of these foods have a bitter taste and therefore offer the perfect antidote to the damp, cool, heavy climate that spring delivers, both internally and externally. Bitter foods are cooling, drying, and light by nature and therefore offer the detoxification support that your body (your liver in particular) needs at this time of year. They also have powerful antibiotic, antiparasitic, and antiseptic qualities. By coordinating your diet with the cycles of the seasons, you effortlessly employ the earth's medicine to help boost your immunity and slough off toxins.

THE CLEANSING DIET

Now that you've given your home and wardrobe a spring cleanse, it's time to do the same for your body. But fear not: you can partake in a spring cleanse on many different levels. You don't need to starve yourself and subsist on water alone! However, if you have never done a cleanse before, I advise you to do it under the professional supervision of an alternative medicine practitioner or an MD who advocates detoxification practices.

The springtime calls us to access the renewing, reparative, and cleansing qualities of plant foods. We can use the medicine of food to clear out what's stagnant and make more space for energy and creativity to emerge again. That means it's time to veer away from winter stews and oatmeal and to start loading up on fruits and vegetables — preferably raw or steamed. After a long winter of consuming the building foods needed to heat and safeguard your body during the colder months, you now need to start eating lighter foods to cleanse, cool, and prepare for the hot days of summer.

At the most basic level, you will need to cut out alcohol, caffeine, red meat, drugs (recreational and unnecessary pharmaceuticals), fried foods, white flour, white sugar, white rice, and dairy — all of which tax the liver, the organ that most needs cleansing this season — for seven to twenty-one days while loading up on fresh fruits, vegetables, and whole grains (and drinking plenty of water, ideally with a squeeze of lemon or a teaspoon of raw apple cider vinegar). The recipes included later in this chapter, as well as the one-day spring cleansing retreat (page 81), will give you some concrete ideas about how to do this. To do this first-stage detox, add herbs such as dandelion and milk thistle — both of which help to cleanse and build the liver.

The next level of cleansing, which I recommend after you have been on the initial cleansing diet for a while (so that you don't experience extreme detox reactions) — is juice feasting. This means having only fresh, raw fruit and vegetable juices for two to seven days. I advise first-timers to start with two to three days. A weekend juice feast, for instance, would be an excellent way to start.

SPRING ALLERGIES

Denise, a New Jersey–based real estate agent, dreads the arrival of spring each year because, for her, it means hay fever. Affecting about forty million people in the United States, its symptoms include sneezing, itchy and watery eyes, a runny nose, sinus congestion, and fatigue.

Barely able to function, much less feel clear and energized enough to feed her creative life and participate in spring's opportunities for expansion, Denise came to one of my retreats, equipped with her tissues and over-the-counter allergy medication. During our afternoon break, she came to me for advice. Having suffered from spring allergies in the past, I suggested what had worked for me, and I offer the same things to you now:

1. Do an elimination diet. First, cut out all dairy for seven days. Dairy creates a lot of mucus in the body and is usually one of the main allergy culprits. I told her to notice how she felt after that first week and then to slowly reintroduce dairy to see how she felt when she did. If the allergies intensified, she should cut it out entirely until her system was strong again. Instead of cow's milk she used almond milk in her cereal and coconut milk in her coffee. Later she had goat cheese or yogurt (easier for human bodies to digest than products made from cow's milk) as occasional treats.
2. Do a supervised juice and colon cleanse. After I did my first one, my allergies completely disappeared.
3. Introduce more omega-3 fatty acids through either fish oil or flaxseed oil capsules or freshly ground flaxseeds each day, which can help reduce allergy-associated inflammation in the body.
4. Engage in some vigorous exercise for twenty to thirty minutes at least three times a week: hiking, biking, flow yoga, fast walking. This helps to induce sweating and to boost circulation, both of which help to strengthen immunity and burn up excessive moisture (including mucus).

A few months later Denise sent me an email thanking me for the suggestions. She had just come back from her first detox retreat, was eating dairy-free, and was feeling brighter and better than ever.

I won't lie: detoxing can be really challenging. You're stripping away one of your greatest comforts and constants: food. Plus, you may be feeling the repercussions of cleansing, from headaches to hunger pangs. Here are a few tips for dealing with this discomfort:

1. Sip hot water throughout the day. Water helps to flush out toxins and to bring a feeling of fullness. Often when we feel hungry, we're really thirsty. Ayurveda recommends a daily practice of sipping hot water to flush debris from tissues.

(continued on next page)

SPRING ALLERGIES *(continued)*

2. Surround yourself with inspiration. Read nutrition and health books. In moments of doubt, you can turn to these to remember why you're doing all this!

3. Cleanse your colon. I know there's a lot of cultural stigma around this one, and the first time I did a detox I (literally) almost passed out when my guide did a mock demonstration of how to do a colonic. But once I tried it, I realized how natural and essential this is to human health. Do some research about colonics and talk to a professional (such as your acupuncturist or naturopath) about whether these would be appropriate for you. If so, find a way to incorporate one into your cleanse — either by doing an at-home enema or by going to a professional for colon hydrotherapy. As toxins are released from your organs, they gather and accumulate in your digestive tract — and your colon in particular. You need some form of colon cleansing to brush these out and help give you a renewed sense of lightness and clarity.

LOVING YOUR LIVER

The liver, which ancients considered the most important organ in the body, is the largest internal organ. Weighing three to four pounds and located in your upper right abdomen, just below your diaphragm, it's rightly named, for your liver's good functioning is crucial to your health. Its duties include producing bile for breaking down fats; storing vitamins A, D, K, and B_{12}, as well as

FOODS TO SUPPORT YOUR LIVER

Emphasize cooling, bitter, and fresh foods to reinvigorate your body and to help your liver rejuvenate from all the hard work it does for you in filtering toxins — from the food, water, and air. Here's a list of some specific foods that can help:

- spirulina, chlorella, and wheatgrass
- dandelion root tea
- burdock root
- sarsaparilla
- Yogi DeTox tea
- lemon juice
- olive oil and olives
- raw apple cider vinegar
- milk thistle seed (tea or extract)
- dark green, leafy vegetables
- steamed and raw foods

other minerals and glycogen; storing blood when you're at rest and releasing it when you spring into activity; filtering toxins from the blood; and distributing nourishment through your body. Anything that can't be broken down and used for energy ends up in the liver for detoxification. When you overindulge in alcohol, chemicals, drugs, fried foods, "white foods" (white flour, dairy, white sugar), and red meat, your liver becomes overworked, unable to detoxify your blood effectively. In the modern world, since so few of us live in pristine and unpolluted environments, it has the added load of being continually barraged by toxins in our air, soil, water, and pesticide-laden foods. Therefore, it's imperative that we cleanse our livers at least once or twice a year for optimal functioning.

The gallbladder, a small sac-shaped organ, rests behind the liver. Here's where the bile from the liver flows to be housed and secreted as needed during digestion. We'll take a closer look at the energetic, mental, and emotional qualities of these two organs in the next chapter.

THINGS TO AVOID TO SUPPORT YOUR LIVER

- overeating
- overly spicy foods
- fried foods
- caffeine (black tea, coffee, soda)

- alcohol
- rich, complicated meals
- overly creamy or sweet foods

Let's take all this information and put it into action. Remember, as a woman, you're a born creator — and that includes being an artist in the kitchen. Use your hands and spring's produce to assemble healing and vibrant meals to nourish you and your family. Grab your cloth shopping bag and head to your local farmers' markets to get started, but don't do it begrudgingly. Delight in the experience. Invite a friend or family member to go with you, and make it an outing. Rather than viewing your shopping and cooking as chores, set aside a few hours for each of these activities, and allow them to be opportunities for interacting and for enjoying the colors, smells, and tastes of the world around you. Let yourself be touched and surprised by what you discover. Gathering and preparing our food is essential for staying alive, so you might as well enjoy it! Also, don't be afraid to ask questions and create relationships with the vendors. This was one of my favorite things about living in Thailand. I shopped mostly at outdoor fruit and vegetable markets and enjoyed seeing the same faces week after week, year after year. If you're not sure what something is, ask! The growers will also often have great tips for how to cook with the more unusual vegetables.

For even more guidance, in each season I'll offer you a shopping list as well as recipes and menu suggestions for breakfast, lunch, dinner, snacks, and desserts.

THE DIRTY DOZEN AND THE CLEAN FIFTEEN

THE DIRTY DOZEN: THE TWELVE MOST CONTAMINATED FOODS (FROM WORST TO BEST)

These foods harbor the most pesticides when grown conventionally. Always buy their organic versions.[1]

1. celery
2. peaches
3. strawberries
4. apples
5. blueberries
6. nectarines
7. bell peppers
8. spinach
9. cherries
10. kale/collard greens
11. potatoes
12. grapes (imported)

THE CLEAN FIFTEEN: THE LEAST CONTAMINATED FOODS (FROM BEST TO WORST)

If need be (because of price or availability), you can get by with eating the nonorganic versions of these:

1. onions
2. avocado
3. sweet corn
4. pineapple
5. mango
6. sweet peas
7. asparagus
8. kiwi
9. cabbage
10. eggplant
11. cantaloupe
12. watermelon
13. grapefruit
14. sweet potato
15. honeydew melon

TRY THIS

If my father ever came to visit me during the spring, he would be appalled! Dandelions — the very things that he diligently mowed from my childhood lawn — reign wild and unbridled. Why? Dandelions come forth each year, bearing the gifts of spring's most potent medicine. A cleansing, bitter tonic for the liver, blood, and kidneys, they also help to clear obstructions in digestive organs and balance digestive enzymes. Head out into your yard this spring and pick some dandelions (but only if you have a chemical-free lawn; otherwise, buy some at the store or local farmers' market) to put in your salads, to add to a stir-fry, to juice them, or to make a healing tea from them.

DANDELION HERB TEA

6 tablespoons dried dandelion root (found at herb shops)
4 cups filtered water
6 tablespoons dried dandelion leaf, or 12 tablespoons fresh dandelion leaf

Simmer dandelion root and leaf in the water, uncovered, for 20 minutes. Strain the liquid into a sealable glass container. Drink immediately or cover tightly and save for later.

SPRING SHOPPING LIST

After a dormant winter, farmers' markets come to life again in the spring. Here are some of the treats that you might find there at this time of year. Remember, now's the time to really load up on anything and everything green!

apples	garbanzo beans	pineapple
artichokes	ginger	quinoa
asparagus	grapefruit	radicchio
avocado	kale	radishes
beets	kiwi	rhubarb
berries	lemons	sassafras
broccoli	lettuce	snow peas
burdock root	limes	spirulina
carrot	milk thistle	sprouts
celery	millet	strawberries
cinnamon	mung beans	Swiss chard
dandelion	onion	Valencia oranges
escarole	parsley	watercress

BREAKFAST REVOLUTION

Let's take these foods now and make art with them, starting with breakfast.

We've all heard it before: breakfast is the most important meal of the day. To ensure that your energy stays steady and strong through this highly productive stretch from waking until lunch, pay special attention to what you eat. Research shows that a balance of protein, healthy fats, and carbohydrates gives us the energy we need while putting minimal strain on our digestive system. Try it out for yourself, and see how your body responds! This means that breakfast foods such as sugar-laden cold cereals, doughnuts, bagels, toast, and pancakes (unless you opt for the gluten- and white sugar–free versions) can throw your body off balance by supplying a sudden burst of energy followed by a crash — which is normally when you reach for extra caffeine or sugar to keep you going until lunch.

For the past decade, my breakfast of choice has been smoothies. This habit started in Thailand, where tropical fruits — papaya, mango, banana, and pineapple — reign. Luckily, the habit stuck, and I find that wherever I am in the world, 99 percent of the time I want a smoothie to start my day. They're easy to prepare, infinitely creative, packed with energy and nutrients, and very gentle on your digestive system. They're also easy to drink on the go, if need be, and they're delicious and a lot of fun to eat (I like to pour mine in a bowl and eat it with a spoon). Kids love them too. Whenever I visit my nephews in Chicago, they always want to drink a smoothie with me, even if the smoothie is green!

On mornings when you want a lighter breakfast, make your smoothie more fruit and vegetable dense. When you're feeling hungrier or in need of more stamina, add more protein. Each season I'll also offer you a nonsmoothie breakfast option if you want to mix things up a little bit.

BREAKFAST MENU

- Cinnamon Amaranth Flax Porridge
- Spring Green Smoothie

CINNAMON AMARANTH FLAX PORRIDGE

Serves 2

Originally from Mexico and a sacred food of the Aztecs, amaranth is higher in protein and calcium than milk, making it especially beneficial for nursing or pregnant women, infants, children, and those who expend a lot of energy through work or exercise. Plus, one bowl contains 60 percent of your daily iron dosage, so it's great to include during menstruation, and it's cooling and astringent, a perfect addition to a spring diet. Flaxseeds and sunflower seeds add some extra fiber and healthy fats. The cinnamon is warming for cool spring mornings and helps to stimulate circulation.

½ cup amaranth
1½ cups filtered water
a pinch of sea salt
¼ teaspoon cinnamon
1 tablespoon flaxseeds
1 small handful sunflower seeds (raw or dry roasted, with a dash of tamari
    for a more savory dish)
maple syrup, agave nectar, or raw honey to taste

Rinse the amaranth and set aside. Place the water in a small saucepan. Add the sea salt and cinnamon and bring to a boil. Once the water is boiling, add the amaranth. Bring to a boil again, turn heat to low, and cover. Cook 30 to 45 minutes. Watch it closely toward the end, since it gets quite gooey and can stick to the bottom of the pan; you may need to stir it. Grind the flaxseeds in a coffee grinder (these seeds go rancid very quickly once exposed to air and light, so it's best to do it fresh). Put the amaranth in a bowl, and garnish with

THE SEASON FOR SEEDS

Spring holds the potential for new life. Think about it: from a tiny acorn an entire oak tree can grow and live for hundreds of years! So much potential is packed into a tiny seed. Spring is a great time to increase your seed intake. To make them easier to digest, soak raw seeds in water overnight, and then drain. Otherwise, buy dry-roasted ones (or dry-roast them yourself). If you're working with your fertility, seeds are a great thing to eat more of too. Makes sense, right?

the ground flaxseeds, sunflower seeds, and maple syrup. You can also add a sugar-free nut milk if you like (recipe on page 150).

TIP: You can also make a larger batch to reheat on subsequent mornings to save time!

SPRING GREEN SMOOTHIE

Serves 1

A delicious way to start your day (while eating your greens for breakfast)!

> 1 large handful frozen or fresh mango pieces
> 1 cup coconut water, almond milk (recipe on page 150), or fresh orange juice
> ½ cup filtered water, plus more as needed
> 1 tablespoon freshly ground flaxseeds
> 1 scoop brown rice protein powder
> 1 teaspoon spirulina
> 4 drops stevia extract or 1 spoonful raw honey (to sweeten)
> 2 big handfuls baby spinach
> 1 celery stalk

Put mango, coconut milk, almond milk, or orange juice, and ½ cup of water in a blender. Add more water if you need to until the ingredients are covered. Blend well. Add the flaxseeds, protein powder, spirulina, and sweetener — plus any other superfoods that you like (see the list below). Add the vegetables, and continue to blend until smooth.

GREEN SMOOTHIES 101

Making green smoothies can be easy and fun. Here's what you need to know to get started:

- The general rule of thumb is to use this equation: 50 percent fruits + 50 percent vegetables. It's best to include one of the following to add creaminess: half a banana, some frozen mango, or a quarter avocado. Bananas will add sweetness, but if the smoothie's not sweet enough, add some fresh juice, coconut water, agave, stevia, or raw honey.
- Blend fruit and liquid first, then add the greens.
- Make homemade popsicles out of any leftover juice or smoothies.
- For an extra kick add some pineapple, turmeric, ginger, lemon, or lime.

- Experiment with different greens to find a combination that suits you. Mix and match some of the following:

arugula
baby greens (spring mix)
baby spinach
barley grass
celery

chard
cilantro
cucumbers
kale
mint
parsley

romaine lettuce
sprouts
wheatgrass
wild greens (such as nettles or dandelion)

THE SUPERFOODS FACTOR

You can also add some high-energy extras to your smoothies to pack in more nutritional power. Generally you would add one scoop of any or all of the superfoods listed below (read the product label for more specific instructions). But be aware that these can drastically alter the taste and texture of your smoothie, so start sparingly until you get it just right and determine what you like.

Generally, you want to include some greens (either in their natural form or as a powder), some fats (coconut oil, avocado, flaxseed oil, chia seeds, or nut butter), and some protein (hemp seed powder, brown rice powder, or nut milk or nut butter) to make your smoothie as balanced and nutritionally dense as possible. Visit www.TheWayoftheHappyWoman.com for details about where to order the ingredients below.

Here's a brief overview of some of my favorite superfoods:

- *Hemp seed powder.* Hemp seed, a great source of protein, is considered one of the most nutritious food sources on the planet.
- *Brown rice protein powder.* Gluten-free and a fantastic alternative to soy, this powder offers a quick, allergy-free way to get extra protein while enjoying the benefits of brown rice.
- *Spirulina.* Spirulina is one of the most nutrient-dense foods on the planet. This blue-green, single-celled algae offers a concentrated source of complete, balanced protein. Spirulina also displays high levels of the antioxidants beta-carotene and zeaxanthin, plus immune-supportive elements found in no other food. This incredible green protein powerhouse also displays potent blood-purification properties, and it is one of the only sources of the anti-inflammatory, joint-strengthening super omega-6 fatty acid GLA (gamma-linolenic).
- *Cacao powder.* Cacao, the pure source of ordinary chocolate, was revered by ancient cultures as the food of the gods. Research now links the antioxidants in

(continued on next page)

THE SUPERFOODS FACTOR *(continued)*

cacao to everything from cardiovascular health to improved brain function and longevity! Cacao even provides the same endorphins our brain makes when we're happy or in love. Cacao powder is also a low-fat way to introduce the health and zing of raw chocolate into your smoothies.

- *Carob powder.* The carob tree is a member of the legume family and grows in Mediterranean areas. Carob has rightly been coined the healthy alternative to chocolate, since it is free of the stimulants caffeine and theobromine found in chocolate. It is also naturally sweet, so carob products will generally contain substantially less sugar than their chocolate counterparts. Carob powder can be substituted for cocoa powder in any recipe. Moreover, carob has up to 8 percent protein and contains vitamins A, B, B_2, B_3, and D. It is also high in calcium, phosphorus, potassium, and magnesium and contains iron, manganese, barium, copper, and nickel.

- *Maca powder.* Maca has been a traditional health and vitality secret since the days of the ancient Inca — and has been revered as a powerful aphrodisiac. Similar to ginseng and other adaptogenic foods, Maca has a potent nutritional content that enhances your ability to balance hormones and handle stress while boosting energy. Try a scoop in your smoothies, juices, and chocolate recipes, and discover for yourself the powerful effects!

- *Goji berries.* With their high antioxidant levels, trace minerals, and eighteen amino acids, goji berries put the *super* in *superfood*, providing cholesterol-reducing phytosterols and eyesight-protecting carotenoids. Blend the powder into smoothies, or in their whole, berry form, put them in your cereal, smoothies, and trail mixes — or just eat them alone as a snack.

- *Mesquite powder.* Mesquite powder has a molasses-like flavor with a slight hint of caramel. Its tastes great in teas, coffees, and smoothies, dairy or seed/nut yogurts, energy bars, and fruit/nut butter spreads. Mesquite is also highly effective in balancing blood sugar. Because its sugar is in the form of fructose, which does not require insulin for metabolism, mesquite helps maintain a sustained blood sugar level. It is useful for diabetics and helps maintain a healthy insulin system in others. Because mesquite powder is ground from the entire pod, including the seed, it is high in protein (11 to17 percent). It is also rich in lysine, calcium, magnesium, potassium, iron, zinc, and fiber.

- *Chia seeds.* Rich in fiber, omega-3 fatty acids, calcium, iron, and protein, the chia seed was eaten by the Aztecs for strength and was a staple food, along with corn and beans. It has much in common with flaxseed, with the distinct advantage that its natural antioxidants make it more stable. Soak the seeds in water first, for about ten to twenty minutes (10 parts water to 1 part seed). Then add some to cereals or smoothies — you can even use them to replace the fats in baked goods. I include some of these (either whole and soaked or as a ground powder) in all my meals. They help to create a feeling of fullness, in addition to providing vital nutrition.

- *Coconut oil.* Coconut oil or butter consists of 90 percent or more of raw, saturated fat — a rare and important building block of every cell in the human body. It is an antimicrobial, supporting the immune system, thyroid gland, nervous system, and skin. It provides fast energy and helps to increase metabolism.

MORE BREAKFAST IDEAS

- Yogi DeTox tea sweetened with raw honey and a slice of toasted Ezekiel bread with almond butter.
- Scrambled eggs with spring onion and parsley, wrapped in a brown rice tortilla with sprouts.
- A quick green detox shake with brown rice protein powder, coconut water, and spirulina or a green powder blend (you can even make it at work by putting everything in a mason jar and shaking it up).

LUNCH MENU

- Kale Salad with Sprouts
- Split Pea Soup

KALE SALAD WITH SPROUTS

Serves 2 to 4

Here's one of my staple dishes, year-round. It's also a crowd-pleaser at potlucks, and you can vary it endlessly. Kale is very hearty and does well throughout most of the year, actually becoming more flavorful after a frost. A wonderful anti-inflammatory, kale is also very rich in calcium, vitamins, and antioxidants.

1 bunch organic kale (I like dinosaur, or Lacinato, kale the best)
2 tablespoons lemon juice

2 tablespoons extra virgin olive oil

1 tablespoon tamari or Bragg's Liquid Aminos

1 tablespoon dulse flakes

1 handful alfalfa sprouts (or your favorite sprouts)

Wash the kale and rip small pieces away from the spines (compost the spines), and place them in a bowl. Use your hands to massage the lemon juice, olive oil, and tamari into the kale. Do this until the leaves are tender. Add the remaining ingredients, toss, and enjoy!

A WORD ABOUT SPROUTING

I used to be afraid of sprouting. Would I *do* it wrong? Would the seeds never grow? Would I forget to water them? When I finally brought myself to actually do it, it was easy! Here's a simple way to get started. We'll start with alfalfa seeds, and then gradually you can go on to sprout seeds, nuts, legumes, and even grains to make delicious raw meals, snacks, and accoutrements. An added nutritional bonus: when you sprout something, its protein content increases, and the food is still living. In fact, it's *more* alive now than it was as a seed, and your body is going to ingest all that life force....

1. Get some quart-size glass jars (I like mason jars) and some screens or sprouting lids. (You can also buy the whole sprouting kit at a conscious hardware/houseware or health food store.)
2. Put 2 tablespoons of alfalfa seeds in the jar, and cover with the screen lid.
3. Rinse the seeds and then fill the jar at least a quarter full with room-temperature water, and let it sit overnight.
4. Remove the water, then roll the jar around to encourage the seeds to stick to the sides.
5. Place the jar on its side, at a 45-degree angle, on a downward slope. You can rest it in a colander or bowl, away from direct sunlight.
6. Rinse the seeds once or twice a day (twice if it's warm outside). Do this by filling the jar with clean water, swishing it around the seeds, then pouring out the water. Repeat step 5.
7. Repeat this for five to six days, until they look like full-grown alfalfa sprouts. Put them in the sun for about fifteen minutes so they get nice and green. Then enjoy! Refrigerate them in a container once they've drained for several hours.

SPLIT PEA SOUP

Serves about 10

This soup adds some nice protein and warmth to your meal for those cool spring days, and if you make a big batch, you can freeze it, which will save you time later. For a heartier version, add some potatoes.

2 tablespoons olive oil

1 small yellow or white onion, chopped

2 bay leaves

2 to 3 small garlic cloves, minced

2 cups dried split peas

1 teaspoon sea salt

2½ cups low-sodium vegetable stock

5 cups water

3 carrots, chopped

3 stalks celery, chopped

1 teaspoon minced fresh thyme leaves (or ½ teaspoon dried)

3 tablespoons coarsely chopped fresh parsley

1 tablespoon tamari

ground black pepper to taste

In a large pot, sauté the oil, onion, bay leaves, and garlic over medium-high heat for 5 minutes, or until onions are translucent. Add the peas, salt, vegetable stock, and water. Bring everything to a boil, reduce heat, and simmer for 2 hours, stirring occasionally. Add the carrots, celery, thyme, parsley (setting aside a little for later), tamari, and pepper. Simmer for another hour, or until everything is tender. Garnish with the remaining parsley, and serve hot.

TIP: Add some cooked millet, brown rice (1 part grain to 1 part water, a dash of sea salt, brought to a boil and simmered for 30 to 40 minutes, until fluffy), or gluten-free bread to this meal. I like the brands Manna Bread and Garden of Life. You can also find great gluten-free bread recipes at www.Elanas Pantry.com.

MORE LUNCH IDEAS

- Steamed broccoli, millet, and tofu drizzled with olive oil, lemon juice, and gomasio.
- Stir-fried spinach, ginger, chickpeas, curry powder, and tamari served over long-grain brown rice.

SNACK MENU

- Hummus
- Beet Chips

HUMMUS

Serves about 6

Hummus is a potent protein source and can be served with whole-grain bread, including pita, or vegetable sticks.

1 teaspoon cumin seeds
2 cups cooked, sprouted, or canned chickpeas (about ½ cup dried chickpeas, soaked overnight and then cooked)
1 clove garlic
¼ cup olive oil, plus more for serving
2 tablespoons fresh lemon juice
1 tablespoon tahini
½ cup parsley plus a few sprigs for garnish
¾ teaspoon sea salt
optional: paprika for garnish

In a small skillet, toast the cumin seeds until they become fragrant (about 2 minutes). According to the Ayurvedic tradition, the healing energy of spices is activated when you roast them. In a food processor, puree the chickpeas and garlic with the cumin, olive oil, lemon juice, tahini, parsley, and salt until smooth and creamy. Add 1 to 2 tablespoons water as necessary to achieve the desired consistency. Transfer to a bowl. Drizzle with olive oil, and, if you like, sprinkle with paprika and/or add a parsley sprig before serving.

BEET CHIPS

Serves about 4

My friend Syda introduced me to this healthy and colorful alternative to the traditional potato chip. These are a potent blood builder — great to eat during menstruation. Even those who don't like beets appreciate them. They make fun hors d'oeuvres too.

4 medium-large beets, scrubbed well (do not peel unless they're not organic)
1 tablespoon olive oil
½ tablespoon tamari
sea salt and black pepper to taste

Preheat oven to 400°F. Slice beets thinly (so they look like potato chips). Put them in a bowl, and toss them with olive oil, tamari, salt, and pepper. Spread them evenly on two cookie sheets, and roast for 45 minutes to an hour, turning halfway through, until crisp. Check often to make sure they don't burn!

DINNER MENU

• Quinoa and Roasted Asparagus Tabouli

CANNED FOODS: TO EAT OR NOT TO EAT?

I have a huge aversion to canned foods. For the most part, I don't think we're meant to eat food that's so far removed from its natural form. However, there are times when canned foods are helpful — when you're in a hurry and want to prepare something healthy that usually takes a long time to cook, as in the case of beans.

That's the reason I usually keep a few cans of no-salt-added, organic beans in my pantry for those moments: garbanzo beans, black beans, and adzuki beans. Just make sure to rinse them well before using them to remove any film they've accumulated from the canning process.

QUINOA AND ROASTED ASPARAGUS TABOULI

Serves 3 to 4

Quinoa, pronounced "keen-wa," was revered by the Incas as their "mother grain." Full of energizing protein and easy to digest, it's strengthening for the whole body and cooks quickly and easily. It's also high in bone-boosting minerals such as copper, phosphorus, iron, and magnesium and is a good source of PMS-fighting manganese. Plus, it is delicious — and makes for a great lunch the next day!

½ cup red or white quinoa (rinsed well)
1 cup water
sea salt
2 tablespoons lemon juice
1 tablespoon balsamic vinegar
2 tablespoons extra virgin olive oil
1 teaspoon agave nectar or raw honey
1 teaspoon tamari or Bragg's Liquid Aminos
1 bunch asparagus, bottoms cut off
1 medium carrot, shredded
2 tablespoons white sesame seeds (raw or toasted)
1 handful raisins
1 spring onion, minced
fresh ground pepper

Preheat the oven to 400°F. Boil quinoa in 1 cup water and a dash of sea salt, then reduce to a simmer for 15 to 20 minutes, until all the water is absorbed. Remove from heat, and let sit for 5 minutes, then fluff with a fork. Whisk together the lemon juice, vinegar, olive oil, agave, and tamari in a small bowl, and set aside. Put asparagus in the oven, and broil for 20 minutes, until browned and tender, or place on the grill on high heat for a few minutes. Remove asparagus from heat and slice into 1-inch pieces. Put quinao, asparagus, carrot, sesame seeds, raisins, and onion in a bowl, and stir in the dressing. Season with sea salt and fresh ground pepper to taste.

OPTIONAL: You can also serve the tabouli over a bed of arugula, baby spinach, and any other fresh greens you like. You can leave the greens dry, to soak in the flavor of the quinoa tabouli, or toss them lightly in My Favorite Salad Dressing (recipe on page 157). Serve warm.

MORE DINNER IDEAS

- Leftover quinoa stir-fried with julienned carrots, watercress, and tempeh (in sesame oil and tamari).
- Brown rice noodles tossed in miso tahini sauce (equal parts miso, tahini, and warm water whisked together) and topped with steamed Swiss chard.

DESSERT MENU

- Raspberry Crisp

RASPBERRY CRISP

Serves 8

This is one of my favorite desserts to make, and it's always a crowd-pleaser. I often use fruit that I've bought in a case (as seconds or slightly damaged) at the farmers' market — such as peaches, pears, berries, or apples. This crisp is a real comfort food that's healthy enough to enjoy for breakfast!

coconut oil for oiling pan
flour for dusting pan

BERRY FILLING
½ cup apple juice or apple cider
1 tablespoon arrowroot powder
6 cups frozen raspberries
¼ teaspoon vanilla extract

TOPPING
1 cup whole rolled oats (if you have gluten sensitivity, make sure they're not processed in a plant that also processes gluten)
1 cup brown rice flour, gluten-free flour mix, or almond flour
¼ teaspoon ground cinnamon

½ teaspoon sea salt
¼ cup melted coconut oil
¼ cup agave nectar

Preheat oven to 350°F. Coat an 8-inch square baking pan with oil and a little bit of flour, and set aside. To make the berry filling: Place apple juice in a mixing bowl. Add arrowroot, and stir to dissolve. Add raspberries (no need to defrost them), and toss gently. Transfer to prepared pan, and set aside. To make the topping: Combine oats, flour, cinnamon, and salt in a large bowl. Rub coconut oil into mixture with your fingers, then drizzle agave while mixing with fork. Distribute evenly over berry filling. Bake 20 to 30 minutes, or until topping is golden and fruit is bubbling. Serve warm.

From the outer world of the farmers' market, your kitchen, and your dining room table, let's step into your inner world — onto your yoga mat and your meditation cushion. We'll look at how to detoxify and revitalize in an even deeper way (the effects of which will be enhanced by your clean and green spring diet!).

REMEMBER

- Load up on fruits and vegetables, especially local, in-season, green ones this season. Favor those with a bitter flavor.
- Go easy on your liver by cutting down on (or eliminating) caffeine, alcohol, drugs, red meats, "white foods," and fried foods.
- Sip on sarsaparilla, dandelion, milk thistle, or Yogi DeTox tea, sweetened with a bit of agave or stevia, throughout the season.
- Savor the colors, smells, and textures of your foods as you shop for, cook, and eat them. Let your senses reawaken with the spring!
- Partake in a spring detox at the level you're ready for.
- Act out of self-love, not rigid discipline.

Chapter 8

ON *the* YOGA MAT
Revitalize and Transform

Margot, an ambitious and fiery redhead from New Zealand, attended one of my workshops in Bali a few years ago. She strutted into the open-air studio, adorned in a fuchsia halter top, carrying her yoga mat in a bag made from an Indian sari. I knew from an email she had sent me the week before that Margot was a workshop junkie. Of course she didn't call herself that, but having been on the yoga and self-help circuit long enough myself, I know one when I see one. Margot travels around, taking workshop after workshop. She's well studied and proficient in various yoga techniques and methods, but also stubborn and defensive when it comes to receiving feedback. She never actually takes a firm stance by applying what she's learned to her day-to-day life. This meandering is a way of avoiding herself and not taking responsibility for her direction. Sure, it's fine for a little while, but long-term it becomes a deep resistance to facing reality head-on.

On the outside Margot looked healthy and strong. Clearly she took good physical care of herself, and she had an advanced yoga practice, but when she introduced herself to me before the class, I looked into her eyes and knew better. Her green eyes appeared dull and listless, as if they led to a gaping void rather than into the sparkles of Margot's soul. I smiled inside because I knew that we had met at the perfect time. In the class that followed I focused on the liver and how to rejuvenate it, both physically and energetically — the very medicine Margot needed to soften her aggression and to bring more direction into her daily life, and, in turn, to bring her sparkle back.

MENTAL AND EMOTIONAL QUALITIES OF THE LIVER AND GALLBLADDER

A healthy liver is a crucial component of realizing true health, for it's responsible for moving chi and blood through your body. If your liver's stagnant, your life force will be too. Because of this, Taoist healers nicknamed the liver "the general of the army." When functioning optimally, the liver is directive and decisive, coordinating the energy flow through your body and communicating with all the different parts to ensure harmony. As women, we can also think of the liver as an inner warrior goddess. She takes charge. When your chi flows freely through your body, unobstructed, you experience a sense of freedom that's felt through spaciousness and an easygoing disposition. Also, since they directly reflect the health of your liver chi, your eyes shine. Liver chi also governs the health of your hands, nails, and feet, as well as your muscles and tendons.

A healthy liver imbues you with the positive qualities of the spring season's dominant wood element, making you feel stable yet flexible while you reach for your dreams, like a deeply rooted tree. And, just as wood grows out of water, to keep this element healthy and in check, you need to pass through the full cycle of each year, especially the stillness and rest of the watery winter season. Avoiding this natural rhythm by trying to live the same way year-round can leave you burned out with erratic, toxic emotions. In fact, well-functioning liver chi assures balanced emotions and an easy premenstrual week.

DETOXING YOUR MIND

In addition to cleansing your home and body this season, also pay some attention to your thoughts. Usually, challenging emotions spring from unsupportive ways of thinking. Practice becoming mindful of your self-talk as you move through your day. Regular yoga (especially the slow, quiet practice of yin yoga) and Mindfulness Meditation will help you get better acquainted with your inner dialogue. Approach your thoughts with curiosity and compassion. You are *not* your thoughts; they are just one dimension of you. In your meditation practice, when thoughts arise, label them by saying to yourself, "thinking," and then return to the anchor of your breath. The goal of meditation is not to stop thinking, but to become the master of, rather than the servant to, your mind. At the end of your practice, write in your journal what you noticed during your sit. Were you obsessed with planning? Fantasizing about the future? Rehashing a painful situation? Without judgment, notice where your mind likes to go.

Throughout your day you can also start to replace negative thoughts with more positive ones (only after you notice what they are so you're not stuffing or denying them). Some of my favorite affirmations include "I love and accept myself as I am," "Everything is working out for my highest good. All is well," "My body is restoring itself to its natural state of balance," "My life is an endless stream of miracles," and "I am surrounded by love, joy, friends, and laughter."

BECOME A POSTURE PRINCESS

People always compliment me on my good posture. I attribute this to my years of ballet training as a girl as well as to my mom's friend, Jeanne, who lived in a studio apartment on New York City's Upper East Side, sold diamonds at Tiffany, and taught me all about good manners, posture included. My yoga and meditation practices have without a doubt helped me to maintain that as I age. Many others report that after starting yoga, they grew an inch or more — evidence that these ancient tools help to create more space and length in your spine.

When coming onto your yoga mat, the position of your spine relative to your pelvis is paramount in determining how your energy will or will not flow throughout the rest of your body. Here's how to sit tall and become a posture princess. Any time you're in a seated position (for meditation or yoga), please follow these steps:

1. Sit down on your yoga mat (or a chair), with legs crossed (if you're in a chair, put your feet flat on the floor). Then place your hands underneath your seat, palms up. Rock forward and back a few times, over your hands. Locate two bony knobs, which are your sitting bones.
2. Feel where you're resting on your sitting bones. If you're rocked toward the back end of them, and if your knees are much higher then your hips (if you're cross-legged), stack some neatly folded blankets underneath you. It doesn't matter how many you use, just as long as there are enough to allow you to sit more toward the front of your sitting bones. This will bring back the natural inward curve of your lower back and take your knees lower than your hips. As a result, your spine can lengthen without a lot of muscular contraction, and the hip flexors in your groin can relax with the downward slope of your thighbones.
3. Feel how this position of your pelvis relaxes your body and allows energy to move more freely.

If you're feeling stuck or paralyzed, you won't be able to bend with the breezes that blow through your branches, as a healthy tree would. When your liver chi is strong, you're clear about your life path and equipped with the inner tools you need to move steadfastly in that direction, overcoming obstacles as they arise with skillfulness and resilience. You're able to assess a situation, make a clear decision and plan, and then put them into appropriate action. You're also able to adapt and change course if plans change midstream. If you're feeling irritated, edgy, and frustrated, however, you aren't able to think, much less plan clearly. You lack a sense of inner spaciousness and stability. Your attention's going every which way, and you don't have a sense of the ground beneath you. This restless confusion often reveals other signs of liver chi imbalances that include timidity, hesitation, rage, resistance, PMS, or, at the other end of the spectrum, suppressed anger.

SPRING YIN YOGA

The yin yoga sequence for the spring season targets the liver and gallbladder meridians. Energetic emissaries to the liver and gallbladder, these meridians not only run through these organs directly, thus enhancing their physical health, but also boost the liver chi to harmonize your emotions and overall energy flow. The liver meridians begin at the tips of your big toes, ascend up the inner lines of your legs, enter your body through the groin, and traverse your liver and gallbladder and into your lungs, throat, and head, finally ending in the eyes. The gallbladder meridians begin at the outer corner of each eye and travel through your neck and down into your liver and gallbladder. Then they travel along the outside of your hip and leg, down to their ending point in your fourth toe. If you pay attention to your sensations during the following practice, you'll feel the yin poses gently stretching those pathways.

Before Beginning: Review the sections "Create a Sacred Space" (page 67) and "Yin Yoga" (page 49).

Intention: To rejuvenate and harmonize your liver and gallbladder meridians, to access your creative power, and to center, ground, and focus.

Total Practice Time: 69 minutes

Full Sequence of Illustrations: Page 109

1. *Check-In and Intention* (2 to 3 minutes): Review these in chapter 3.
2. *Vitality Breathing* (2 to 5 minutes): Sit cross-legged on your mat and close your eyes. Rest your palms on your midthighs. Soften your body, and bring your attention to your natural breath. As you inhale, follow your breath all the way down into your belly. If you can't feel it travel there, imagine it moving that low. Where your attention goes, energy flows. This is your power center, your creative home, your womb. As you exhale, imagine energy resting there, like water pooling in a lake. Do this for 2 to 5 minutes. Use this same breath concentration throughout the practice to rejuvenate and ground your precious life force.
3. *Wide-Knee Child's Pose* (5 minutes): Uncross your legs and come into a kneeling position, with your hips resting on your heels. Now open your

SPRING YIN YOGA SEQUENCE

1. Check-In
and Intention

2. Vitality Breathing

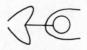

3. Wide-Knee
Child's Pose

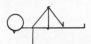

4. Sphinx or Seal Pose

5. Shoelace or Eye of the Needle Pose

6. Shoelace Pose
with Side Stretch

7. Pigeon or Eye of the Needle Pose

8. Dragonfly Pose

9. One-Knee Spinal
Twist

10. Supine Butterfly
Pose

11. Loving-
Kindness Meditation

12. Dedication
of Merit

knees as wide as they're willing to go, keeping your big toes touching. Come forward now, so that your belly rests between your inner thighs, arms stretched overhead along the side of your face, palms down. Rest your forehead on the ground. If that's too far to go, place a pillow or rolled blanket underneath your forehead. At the end of the 5 minutes, slide your inner thighs together and rest for a moment in traditional Child's Pose, then slowly slide your hands under your shoulders and press yourself back upright, so you're sitting on your heels. Now slide your hands forward and lie down on your belly.

4. *Sphinx* or *Seal Pose* (5 minutes): On your belly, place your legs hip width apart and prop yourself up on your elbows, so that they rest slightly in front of your shoulders. Align your forearms so they're parallel, palms down or joined together in prayer position. Keep the back of your neck long, and focus your eyes downward, lowering your eyelids halfway and relaxing your gaze. Feel as if your spine drops through your body toward your belly like a hammock, while your shoulders roll back. For a more advanced variation, put a blanket or cushion under your elbows and clasp each hand to the opposite elbow to give you more height. This will put more pressure on your lower back, so only go for it if you're feeling stable there.

   The most advanced option is to come up into Seal Pose. Press up onto your hands, placing them shoulder width apart, slightly in front of you (the farther out in front of you they are, the less strain will be placed on your lower spine). Turn your hands out slightly, like a seal's flippers. Keep the neck and shoulder positioned as before, in Sphinx Pose. To come out, gently come forward, lengthening your spine on the way down, and rest your forehead on top of your stacked palms. *Note:* If you have any instability in your lower back, slightly contract your lower belly, inner thighs, and outer buttocks.

   Now press back into Child's Pose by placing your hands under your shoulders and inhaling up onto your hands and knees and exhaling as you take your hips back to rest on your heels, big toes touching, arms stretched out overhead. Take several breaths. Now place your hands under your shoulders and press yourself upright so that you're sitting on your heels again.

5. *Shoelace* or *Eye of the Needle Pose* (5 minutes on each side): For Shoelace Pose, swing your hips to one side, coming off your heels and sitting on the floor. Swing your legs around in front of you, and cross your right knee on top of your left, your feet folding back alongside your outer hips. If that's too challenging, keep your left leg straight, with your right leg bent and your knees stacked. Sit up on a blanket if you need the support to keep your spine long. If you're more flexible in your hips, you can inch your feet farther away from your pelvis until your shins become more parallel with the top, short end of your yoga mat. Stay upright if you're feeling a lot of sensation already; otherwise, fold forward, extending your front and back body over your crossed legs. Rest your head on your knee or a

pillow, or put your elbows on the ground and rest your head in the palms of your hands.

If Shoelace Pose feels too difficult for you (especially if you have a knee injury), a wonderful alternative is Eye of the Needle Pose (5 minutes on each side): Lie down on your back and draw your knees in toward your chest. Now cross your right ankle over your left thigh, just above your knee. Weave your left hand to hold behind your left thigh, and your right hand in the space between your thighs to meet it. Use your right elbow to gently coax your right knee away from you, until you feel just the right amount of sensation in your outer right hip, as you use your hands to counteract that by drawing your left knee in toward your chest. Keep your right foot relaxed unless your have a knee injury or sensitivities, in which case you will want to keep it flexed. Breathe deeply. Now switch to the other side. When you've finished, roll to one side and come to rest in Child's Pose.

6. *Shoelace Pose with Side Stretch* (2 minutes on each side): From Shoelace Pose, lean to your right and put your right hand down on the ground. Inhale and lift your left arm. Exhale and bend over to the side, stretching your left arm to the right. You can bend at the elbow and rest your arm on your head. For a deeper stretch along your left side, bring your right hand farther away from your body and bend the elbow without uprooting your hips. Spend a couple of minutes here, and then come to the other side.

7. *Pigeon* or *Eye of the Needle Pose* (5 minutes on each side): From Shoelace Pose, come up onto your hands and knees. Slide your right knee forward so that it lands just behind your right wrist. Slide your left leg back behind you until it lengthens. Let the top of your left thigh rest on the ground and your toes stretch out straight behind you. If you find that you're tipping over to the right, place a rolled blanket or a cushion underneath your right hip to keep your pelvis level. Inhale here, and then exhale and come forward — stopping on your forearms, resting your head in your palms, or coming all the way down with your belly on your front leg and your arms stretched out overhead.

If this puts too much pressure on your front knee or feels too difficult, please do the Eye of the Needle Pose as described in step 5. To come out, inhale and come up; exhale back into Child's Pose. Now go back and repeat Shoelace Pose, Shoelace Pose with Side Stretch, and Pigeon Pose on your left side. When you've finished, come to Child's Pose for 3 to 5 breaths.

8. *Dragonfly Pose* (5 minutes): From Child's Pose, place your hands under your shoulders and push yourself upright to sit on your heels. Swing your hips to the floor on one side of you, and then open your legs into a wide V. Relax your feet. Stay here, or fold forward to the degree that feels comfortable for you. To come out, grip your thighs with your hands and draw your legs back together. Gingerly, lie down on your back, hugging your knees in toward your chest. *Note*: For cases of sciatica or hamstring injuries, please bend your knees slightly and place your feet flat on the ground.

9. *One-Knee Spinal Twist* (5 minutes on each side): With your knees in toward your chest, extend your left leg straight along the ground and hold your right knee with your left hand. Stretch your right arm out on the floor beside you, perpendicular to your body. Inhale here and then exhale, drawing your knee over to the left. If it feels okay for your neck, turn to look over your right hand. Make sure your legs are relaxed. You can use your right hand as a weight on top of your left thigh or use a cushion or blanket under your right thigh and knee if they don't easily touch the floor. As much as possible, keep both shoulder blades on the ground.

    To come out, return to center, drawing your knees in toward your chest. Repeat on the other side. *Advanced students:* For the right side, cross your left thigh over your right, and tuck your left food behind your right calf to form "eagle legs." Repeat on the other side.

10. *Supine Butterfly Pose* (5 to 10 minutes): Lie down on your back. Place the soles of your feet together, your knees open wide so there's a diamond shape inside your legs. If you need support under your knees, roll up two blankets and place one underneath each thigh. Rotate your palms so they face up, a little way away from your hips. Cover up with a blanket if you'd like. Close your eyes, or place an eye pillow over them. Let your whole body relax. Rest deeply, in stillness.

    To come out, begin deepening your breath. Then wiggle your fingers and toes. Roll over onto your right side, and draw your knees in toward your chest. Use your hands to press you up to a seated position. Make your transition slow, smooth, and mindful, and resist jumping up and rushing back into your day.

11. *Loving-Kindness Meditation* (10 to 30 minutes): Cross your legs (the other leg on top now), and follow the meditation instructions at the end of this chapter. You could also begin your yoga practice with a meditation. See what works best for you.

12. *Dedication of Merit* (1 minute): Please review this on page 52.

A MINI-SPRING YIN PRACTICE

Short on time? String these three poses together for a twenty-minute practice. Try them during your lunch break, as your child naps, before your morning shower, or just before sleep.

1. Shoelace or Eye of the Needle Pose
2. Sphinx or Seal Pose
3. Dragonfly Pose

SPRING FLOW YOGA

This practice complements the yin sequence. After having accessed and fed your creative power center, now you will spread that vital energy throughout your body during a heating, detoxifying, and invigorating flow — perfect for clearing away any lingering stuckness or heaviness.

Before Beginning: Review the sections "Create a Sacred Space" (page 67) and "Yang (or Flow) Yoga" (page 50).

Intention: To develop an alert attention, break through resistance and lethargy, warm the body, stimulate the circulatory/respiratory/digestive/lymphatic systems, aid with detoxification, and build core and upper-body strength.

Total Practice Time: 60 minutes

Full Sequence of Illustrations: Pages 114–17

1. *Check-In and Intention* (2 to 5 minutes): Please revisit chapter 3 for details.

2. *Victorious Breathing* (2 minutes): Sit cross-legged, with your palms on your thighs. Keep your eyes open, soft, and downward cast. Gently tone your

SPRING FLOW YOGA SEQUENCE

1. Check-In
and Intention

2. Victorious
Breathing

3. Cow Pose

Cat Pose

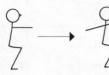

4. Cow Pose with
Leg Lifts

Cat Pose with
Leg Lifts

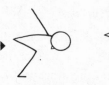

5. Bird Dog Pose

6. Active Child's
Pose

7. Downward-Facing
Dog

8. Standing
Forward Fold

9. Mountain Pose

10. Breath of Joy

11. Mountain
Pose

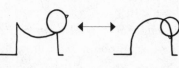

12. Spring Sun
Salutations
*(3 rounds
each side)*

Chair Pose

Clasped-Hand Standing
Forward Fold

Low Lunge

Downward-Facing
Dog

Plank Pose

Push-Ups

SPRING FLOW YOGA SEQUENCE *(CONTINUED)*

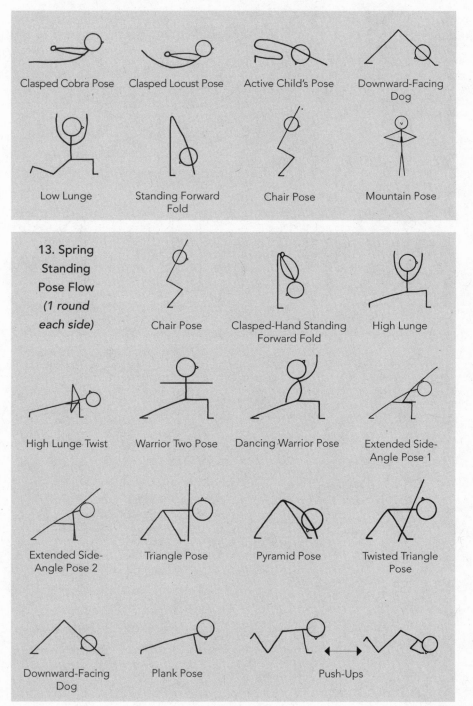

Clasped Cobra Pose

Clasped Locust Pose

Active Child's Pose

Downward-Facing Dog

Low Lunge

Standing Forward Fold

Chair Pose

Mountain Pose

13. Spring Standing Pose Flow *(1 round each side)*

Chair Pose

Clasped-Hand Standing Forward Fold

High Lunge

High Lunge Twist

Warrior Two Pose

Dancing Warrior Pose

Extended Side-Angle Pose 1

Extended Side-Angle Pose 2

Triangle Pose

Pyramid Pose

Twisted Triangle Pose

Downward-Facing Dog

Plank Pose

Push-Ups

SPRING FLOW YOGA SEQUENCE *(CONTINUED)*

Bow Pose

Active Child's Pose

Downward-Facing Dog

Standing Forward Fold

Chair Pose

Mountain Pose

Repeat on other side

Standing Wide-Angle Forward Fold

L-Shaped Handstand

L-Shaped Handstand (Advanced)

Clasped-Hand Standing Forward Fold

14. Floor Flow

Seed Pose

Core Power Bicycle

Core Power Wide-Leg Curl-Ups

Wide Legs

Closed Legs

Bridge Pose

Wide-Legged Bridge Pose

Constructive Rest Pose

Seed Pose

Active Spinal Twist

Seed Pose

SPRING FLOW YOGA SEQUENCE *(CONTINUED)*

Happy Baby Pose

Final Relaxation

15. Loving-Kindness
Meditation

16. Dedication
of Merit

throat muscles, so that your breath makes a soft aspirated sound on both your inhalations and exhalations. It should sound like the ocean when you take a big seashell and hold it up to your ear. With each breath, draw your attention inward. Let this breath focus you and bring you to a more alert, undistracted awareness. When thoughts arise, keep returning to the sound and feeling of your breath. Just as you did in the spring yin sequence, continue the visualization of following your inhale in and down to your pelvis, and on the exhale, feel it rest, widen, and expand there. Use this breath throughout the practice.

Note: If you're menstruating, pregnant, or perimenopausal, don't do the Victorious Breath — you don't need to introduce any more heat to your body now. Just stay with a soft, natural breath, keeping your abdomen relaxed. *Beginners:* Stay with the basic breath outlined in the spring yin yoga sequence.

THE BREATH ENVELOPE

Your breath creates the underlying rhythm of flow yoga. Begin inhaling, and let your movement follow in the wake of your breath. For example, from a standing position, inhale and sweep your arms out to your sides, and at the end of the inhalation, let them reach the end of their range of motion so that your biceps are next to your ears, palms facing each other. Now exhale, and then let your arms retrace their path and land resting by your hips at the end of the exhalation. Always let your breath lead the way and surround the entire experience — from the beginning of the inhalation to the very end of the exhalation — with the envelope of your bare attention.

This simple practice alone can greatly soothe your nervous system — while preventing you from getting injured (it causes you to pay more attention to what you're doing). It's what distinguishes a spiritual embodiment practice from mindless exercise.

3. *Cat/Cow Pose* (5 to 10 rounds): Slide your hands forward, and come onto your hands and knees. Inhale and lift your tailbone and chin toward the ceiling, arching like a cow with her udders stretching toward the earth. Look up toward the space between your eyebrows. As you exhale, swing your tailbone down to point toward the floor beneath your knees. Tuck your chin in toward your chest, arching like a Halloween cat. Move back and forth between these two shapes, following your breath.

4. *Cat/Cow Pose with Leg Lifts* (3 rounds on each side): Inhale into a neutral position of the spine. Exhale and settle there. Inhale and lift your right leg behind you, keeping your hips on the same level and stretching your chest forward, looking up. Exhale and tuck the knee in toward your chin as you round into cat pose. Repeat 3 times and then move onto the other side.

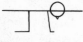

5. *Bird Dog Pose* (5 breaths on each side): Now return to a neutral spine. Gently draw your navel in toward your spine, and as you inhale, lift your left arm and stretch it forward, along your ear, as you stretch your right leg back behind you. Flex your right foot and keep it at the same level as your hips, hugging in toward your midline. Repeat on the other side.

> *Note:* If any of these postures strain your wrists (or you have a wrist injury), either make fists with your hands or do this with your forearms on the ground, parallel, palms flat on the mat.

6. *Active Child's Pose* (3 to 5 breaths): Keeping your toes curled under, sit your hips back on your heels in Child's Pose, with arms stretched overhead, and place your forehead on the ground. Lift your underarms and forearms up toward the ceiling as you stretch your widened palms and fingers down and forward along your mat.

7. *Downward-Facing Dog* (5 breaths): From Child's Pose, inhale back up onto your hands and knees, and on the exhale, lift your hips up and back into Downward-Facing Dog.

8. *Standing Forward Fold* (5 breaths): Mindfully walk your feet up toward your hands until they're directly below your hips and hip width apart.

Place your hands on the floor and sway side to side. Shake your head "yes" and "no" to release your neck.

Note: During standing forward bends (such as Downward-Facing Dog and Standing Forward Fold), feel free to bend your knees as much as you need to in order to release pressure in the backs of your thighs or your lower back. Remember, this isn't about perfection; it's about taking care of yourself and feeling good!

9. *Mountain Pose* (5 breaths): Bend your knees, and keep your fingertips and the crown of your head heavy as your roll yourself up to standing. Drop your weight down evenly through both legs (hip width apart) and feet (balanced on the mound of big toe, baby toe, and center of your heel). Place your hands in front of your heart. *Beginners:* Keep the outer edges of your feet parallel, outer hip width apart. If you have any lower-back sensitivity, come up with a flat back, hands on your hips. *Advanced students:* Bring your feet together, the mounds of the big toes touching, heels slightly apart.

10. *Breath of Joy Pose* (5 times): To stimulate circulation, bend your knees and, without lifting your feet off the ground, bounce gently through your knees as if you were on a trampoline. Briskly inhale and sweep your arms

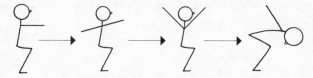

up in front of you, shoulder height, then briskly exhale and lower them to your sides. Briskly inhale and take them out horizontally, then exhale and lower. Inhale and sweep them all the way up toward the sky, then exhale and sweep them down by your sides as you drop your torso forward to rest on your deeply bent knees. Gently smile. Increase the speed as you go. *Note:* For a demonstration of this, please visit www.TheWayoftheHappy Woman.com.

11. *Mountain Pose* (5 breaths): See step 9.

12. *Spring Sun Salutations* (3 rounds): As you do these, visualize the sun coming into you as you inhale, and as you exhale, see the sunlight spreading through and warming you. For the first 2 rounds (each round includes

doing the left and right sides), hold each pose for 5 breaths. For the final round, move through each pose on one breath.

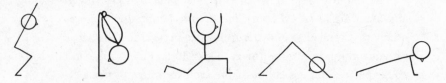

- *Chair Pose:* From Mountain Pose, exhale and bend your knees, then inhale and sweep your arms up next to your ears.

  Beginners: Keep your arms shoulder width apart, palms facing each other. *Advanced students:* Keep your arms straight and place your palms together above your head.
- *Clasped-Hand Standing Forward Fold:* Interlace your fingers behind your back, inhale and open your chest, and exhale as you fold forward.
- *Low Lunge:* Release your hands, step your right leg back, and lower the knee to the ground as you exhale. Inhale and lift your arms up next to your ears.
- *Downward-Facing Dog:* Exhale. Release your arms down to the ground and step back into Downward-Facing Dog.
- *Plank Pose:* Inhale. Glide your shoulders forward over your wrists so that your body forms a long line from the back of your head to your heels. Hollow your belly up toward your spine.

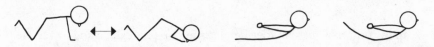

- *Push-Ups* (5 rounds): Do this with your knees up or down. Exhale to lower down, and inhale to come up. Lower down only to the degree to which you can keep your belly drawing in toward your back (rather than sagging through your middle like a tired horse). Bend your elbows back toward your rib cage (rather than out to your sides as in the military). On the sixth round, lower all the way down to your belly.
- *Clasped Cobra Pose* and *Clasped Locust Pose:* Stretch your legs back behind you, hip width apart, and interlace your fingers behind your back. 1) Inhale. Roll your shoulders away from the ground, and on the next inhale, lift your chest up. Hold for 5 breaths. 2) Staying up, also lift your legs, keeping them hip width apart. Hold for 5 breaths. Then slowly lower down.

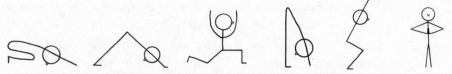

- *Active Child's Pose:* Place your hands under your shoulders, and exhale as you press back into Active Child's Pose.
- *Downward-Facing Dog:* Exhale into it.
- *Low Lunge:* As you exhale, step your right leg forward and lower the left knee to the ground. On the inhale, lift up your arms.
- *Standing Forward Fold:* Inhale and step your back leg forward; exhale as you fold forward.
- *Chair Pose:* Inhale into it.
- *Mountain Pose:* Exhale into it.

Repeat again, this time stepping the left leg back first. Now you've completed your first round. Do one more round (right and left) holding each pose for 5 breaths. Then do a final round (right and left) moving through each pose on one breath — for a total of 3 rounds.

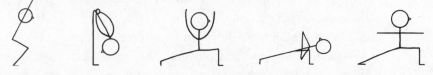

13. *Spring Standing Pose Flow* (hold each of these for 5 to 10 breaths)
    - *Chair Pose:* Inhale into it.
    - *Clasped-Hand Standing Forward Fold:* Exhale into it, with hands clasped behind your back.
    - *High Lunge:* Inhale and step your left leg back. Exhale and pause. Then inhale and lift your arms up overhead, keeping your back heel and knee up.
    - *High Lunge Twist:* Inhale, then exhale and place your palms together in front of your heart in prayer position. On your next exhale, twist your torso to the right, hooking your elbow on the outside of your right thigh. *Beginners:* Lower your back knee down to the ground, if that helps to stabilize you. *Advanced students:* Bring more of your tricep (rather than your elbow) to the outside of your thigh, and then place your left hand on the floor to the outside of your right foot while stretching your right arm up to the sky.
    - *Warrior Two Pose:* Inhale up out of the twist keeping your front knee bent, exhale and pause, then inhale and open your hips to the left side

with your arms out to the sides. Lower the back heel to the ground, so that the foot is at an angle, with the heel farther behind you than the toes. Line up the front heel with the center of the back arch.

- *Dancing Warrior Pose:* From Warrior Two Pose, inhale and slide your left hand down the outside of your back thigh as you arch over to your left and sweep your right arm up alongside your face. Look up if it feels okay for your neck. Exhale, keeping a deep bend in your right knee.

- *Extended Side-Angle Pose:* From Dancing Warrior Pose, inhale back up to Warrior Two and then exhale, bringing your right forearm down to rest on the top of your right thigh. Inhale and sweep your left arm overhead, in line with your left leg. Look forward or up. *Advanced students:* Place your right hand on the floor to the outside of your right knee.

- *Triangle Pose:* From Extended Side-Angle Pose, inhale, and then exhale as you slowly straighten your right knee, keeping it lined up just over your second and third toes. Maintain a tiny bend in your right knee as you place your right hand on your shin (or on a block behind your right shin). Inhale and stretch your left arm up. Look straight ahead or up.

- *Pyramid Pose:* From Triangle Pose, exhale and swivel your hips so they're square over your right foot. Step your back foot forward about a foot, and angle the toes out slightly. Keep your legs hip width apart. With your hands on the floor or on blocks on either side of your front foot, inhale and look forward. Keeping a long spine, exhale and slowly start to reach your chest toward your front shin.

- *Twisted Triangle Pose:* From Pyramid Pose, inhale and look up, keeping your hips square and your feet where they are. With your left hand on the floor, or with the block on the inside of your right foot, exhale and slowly twist your torso over to the right. Inhale and look straight ahead or up. *Beginners:* Keep your right elbow bent, and rest your hand on your lower back as you focus on twisting your spine to the right. *Advanced students:* Place your left hand on the floor on the outside of your right foot, and stretch your right arm up toward the sky.

- *Downward-Facing Dog:* Exhale into it.
- *Plank Pose:* Inhale into it.
- *Push-Ups* (5 rounds): On the sixth round, lower all the way down to the ground.
- *Bow Pose:* Lying on your belly, inhale to reach back and hold the outside of each foot with your hands. Exhale and soften. As you inhale, press your feet back into your hands and lift your chest. Reach your inner heels up to the ceiling as you balance on your pubic bone. Stay here for 5 to 10 breaths, or roll slightly forward and back with your breath to massage your liver. Lower down slowly and rest on your belly for 5 to 10 breaths. Repeat two more times. *Note:* If this feels uncomfortable, place a blanket underneath you for this pose. Beginners can put a strap around each ankle to help reach the feet.
- *Active Child's Pose:* Exhale into it.
- *Downward-Facing Dog:* Exhale into it.
- *Standing Forward Fold:* Exhale into it.
- *Chair Pose:* Inhale into it.
- *Mountain Pose:* Exhale into it.

Repeat the Standing Flow, stepping the right leg back now, and move through the standing flow with the left leg forward. Finish in Downward-Facing Dog.

- *Standing Wide-Angle Forward Fold:* From Downward-Facing Dog, inhale and step your right foot forward between your hands. Walk your hands to your left until they're centered under your chest, and pivot your feet to the left, so your toes are pointing in the same direction as your fingers. Keep your feet about one leg's length apart, and turn your toes in slightly. Inhale extend your spine forward. Exhale and fold forward. To come out, exhale and take your hands to your hips. Inhale and slowly rise.
- *L-Shaped Handstand* (10 to 30 breaths): Bring your mat over to a wall. Sit down with your back against the wall, and stretch your legs straight out in front of you. Notice where your feet are — that's

where you will put your hands. Now, place your hands where your feet were, and come onto your hands and knees, with your hands under your shoulders and knees under your hips, and your backside facing the wall. Spread your fingers really wide, and press down with your fingertips and the base of your fingers. Keep your hands shoulder distance apart. As you inhale, lift your knees up and come into Downward-Facing Dog. Stay here, or slowly start to walk your feet up the wall behind you until they form a 90-degree angle with your torso. *Advanced students:* Lift one leg at a time from the L-Shaped Handstand and hold each side for 10 breaths. After that, you can do a full handstand at the wall or in the center of the room.

- *Clasped-Hand Standing Forward Fold* (5 breaths).

14. *Floor Flow*
    - *Seed Pose:* Lie down on your back, and draw your knees in to your chest. Keep your pelvis on the ground. Interlace your hands over the tops of your shins. Relax your feet. Stay here for 5 to 10 breaths.
    - *Core Power:* With your knees still pulled in to your chest, keep drawing your abdominals in throughout the three following sequences, your lower back pressing into your mat:
        - *Bicycle* (30 to 100 rounds): Interlace your fingers behind your head. Lengthen your right leg out, bend your left knee into your chest, and curl your right elbow up to the outer left knee. Repeat on the other side, and go back and forth. Exhale to come up, and inhale to transition. *Beginners:* Bring the extended leg higher off the ground to make this less intense. *Advanced students:* Bring that leg closer to the ground, and really work on bringing that same shoulder blade fully off the ground as you curl up toward your bent knee.
        - *Wide-Leg Curl-Ups* (30 to 100 rounds): Draw your knees to your chest and take a few rest breaths. Now straighten your legs, soles of feet pointing toward the ceiling, and open your

legs wide apart. Flex your toes back toward your ankles. Exhale, and curl up between your legs, reaching your arms through. If your neck needs more support, place your hands behind your head.

- ◆ *Wide Legs* to *Closed Legs* (7 to 10 breaths): Place your hands on the inside of each thigh, giving a little pressure. Resist your inner thighs into the touch of your hands, as if your legs are trying to close and your hands are preventing that. Let your legs gradually win as you slowly draw them together. It should tax your inner thighs as you go, causing them to quiver slightly. Keep your low back and pelvis on the ground. When you've finished, draw your knees into your chest.

- • *Bridge Pose* (5 to 10 breaths)
  - ◆ Place your feet on the ground, under your knees, hip width apart. Inhale and lift your hips and spine. Walk your shoulders underneath you, and clasp your hands together. Keep your chin and forehead level. *Advanced students:* Just as you did in the L-Shaped Handstand, lift one leg at a time, holding each side for about 5 breaths. To come out, unclasp your hands and slowly roll down from upper to lower back, finally placing your sacrum back on the ground.

  - ◆ Now walk your feet to the outer edges of your mat, keeping them parallel and your knees moving out toward your baby toes. Inhale up into a Wide-Legged Bridge Pose. Hold for 5 to 10 breaths, and slowly lower down.

- • *Constructive Rest Pose* (5 to 10 breaths): Let your inner knees touch while your feet are hip width apart. Rest here for a few breaths. Place both hands on your lower belly. Breathe into your hands.

- • *Seed Pose* (5 breaths).
- • *Active Spinal Twist* (5 times on each side): Take your arms out to your sides in a T position, with your palms facing up. As you exhale, drop

your knees to the right and look to the left. Keep the feet and the inner thighs together, and don't let your knees touch the ground. Inhale up and over to the other side. When you've finished, draw your knees into your chest.

- *Seed Pose* (5 breaths).
- *Happy Baby Pose* (5 to 10 breaths): Lift your feet off the ground so that the soles of your feet point up toward the ceiling and your knees are bent. Keep a 90-degree angle between your thighs and shins. Hold on to the inner edge of each foot with your hands. Actively draw your knees down toward the outside of your rib cage, keeping your pelvis on the ground.
- *Final Relaxation* (5 to 10 minutes): Stretch your legs out so they're a little wider than hip width apart. Let your feet flop out to the sides. Rotate your hands so the palms face up, about a foot away from your hips. Cover up with a blanket if you'd like. Close your eyes, or place an eye pillow over them. Let your whole body relax. Rest deeply, in stillness.
- To come out, begin deepening your breath. Then wiggle your fingers and toes. Roll over onto your right side, and draw your knees in toward your chest. Use your hands to press you up to a seated position. Make your transition slow, smooth, and mindful, and resist jumping up and rushing back into your day.

15. *Loving-Kindness Meditation* (5 to 30 minutes): See page 127.
16. *Dedication of Merit* (1 minute): Please review instructions on page 52.

MINI-SPRING FLOW PRACTICE

If you're short on time, you can do this sequence in fifteen to thirty minutes.

1. Cat/Cow Pose (5 times)
2. Spring Sun Salutations (1 to 3 complete rounds)
3. Bridge Pose (5 breaths)
4. Active Spinal Twist (3 times)
5. Happy Baby Pose (5 breaths)
6. Final Relaxation (2 to 5 minutes)

LOVING-KINDNESS MEDITATION

The more we live from the inside out, in harmony with the seasons of our hearts and lives, the more our innate human qualities can express themselves effortlessly. These include loving-kindness, compassion, joy, and equanimity — what the Buddha called the four heavenly abodes, or your "best home." Expressing these qualities makes you feel most at home in yourself.

Everyone has these four qualities. You don't need to learn them; you just need to remember to dust them off regularly. Doing so reconnects you with your basic goodness. Each season's meditation will offer you the opportunity to focus on one of these abodes, both on your meditation cushion and in your day-to-day life.

The first of these meditations focuses on loving-kindness. Several years ago, while I was working with my meditation mentor, we decided to spend a full year going through each of these four heavenly abodes. However, that year we never got past loving-kindness! Inspired by Jack Kornfield, one of my favorite Buddhist teachers (he also lived in Chiang Mai, as a monk, for many years) who teaches this meditation often, I decided to keep my focus on loving-kindness, for I felt the need to cultivate self-love and self-acceptance, qualities that had been sorely missing in my life. Once I felt grounded enough in the practice that I could authentically offer loving-kindness to myself, I began to practice sending it out to others — family members, friends, benefactors, taxi drivers, and eventually people whom I had been estranged from. I ended up doing this for a full twelve months. When I was talking on the phone, typing emails, or walking down the street, I'd often say to myself, "May I be happy," or "May you be happy," or "May all beings be happy." These simple phrases can make a huge difference in your mood and the quality of your everyday interactions, keeping you from spiraling into negative, stressful thinking.

The Buddha revealed that doing Loving-Kindness Meditation brings good dreams and builds an air of protection around you wherever you go. In fact, he called loving-kindness "the greatest protection in all the world." Other benefits of loving-kindness include increasing self-acceptance, feeling interconnected with others, developing gratitude for those who have supported you, and cultivating forgiveness. The felt sense of kindness generated from this practice is also associated with liver chi harmony because it helps to quell anger (only after you've felt and owned it fully) and nurture warmth. Here's how to practice Loving-Kindness Meditation:

1. *Mindfulness Meditation.* Spend about five minutes following the Mindfulness Meditation practice on page 44. *Note:* If your body and mind feel comfortable and at peace, proceed to the following steps. If not, stay with step 1. You can do the full practice again another time when you're less agitated.

2. *Loving-Kindness Meditation for Yourself.* Now let your attention shift from your breath to the phrases below. In your mind's eye, envision your happiest self, or you as a small child, standing in the sun, smiling back at you. Repeat the following phrases silently to yourself, over and over. You are welcome to personalize them, but don't make them so complicated that you won't remember them! Try reciting these when you're looking at yourself in the mirror while brushing your teeth, driving, making the bed, or walking down the street. Be creative, and know that you can literally practice them anywhere and at any time. *Note:* It doesn't matter what you are feeling inside when you do this. Don't think that you are doing something wrong if you don't feel openhearted during this. The practice has a power of its own. Stay with it. Trust in it.

   May I be filled with loving-kindness.
   May I be safe from inner and outer dangers.
   May I be healthy in body, heart, and mind.
   May I be happy and free.

3. *Loving-Kindness for a Loved One.* Call to mind someone you love dearly. It could be a family member, spouse, child, or benefactor. See her smiling back at you in your mind's eye as the happiest and healthiest version of herself. Recite the following phrases to her, as if you were speaking to her directly. If it helps to use her name, you are welcome to do that. *Note:* There's no rush to move on to this step. As I did, you can spend quite some time on giving loving-kindness to yourself. Only when you truly love yourself can you open to loving others.

   May you be filled with loving-kindness.
   May you be safe from inner and outer dangers.
   May you be healthy in body, heart, and mind.
   May you be happy and free.

4. *Loving-Kindness for a Neutral Person.* Think back to a time in your recent past when you encountered someone new: the bus driver, the cashier at the coffee shop, the person who rode the elevator with you. Choose someone you don't know personally and have no ties with. Imagine him smiling back at you in your mind's eye, and recite for him the same four phrases.

5. *Loving-Kindness for an Enemy.* Recall a person you've been challenged by. Maybe you had a falling-out ten years ago. Perhaps you have some bitterness toward your recent ex. Bring him or her to your mind's eye, smiling back at you, and recite the phrases of loving-kindness. *Note:* Don't move on to this step until the previous ones feel fluid and natural. Stay with this one as long as you need to, over time, until it doesn't feel charged. Allow yourself to feel whatever you feel as you move through the practice.

6. *Loving-Kindness for All Beings.* Recite the four phrases below to the people in your home; on your street, in your town, city, state, region, country, hemisphere; and then all across the planet. Feel out in all directions, excluding no one. Include all the creatures of the land, air, and sea. Hug them all to you with these phrases. Feel your connection to them. Embrace them all as a generous mother would.

   May all beings be filled with loving-kindness.
   May all beings be safe from inner and outer dangers.
   May all beings be healthy in body, heart, and mind.
   May all beings be happy and free.

7. *Conclusion.* To finish your practice, return to the Mindfulness Meditation for a minute or two. Then bring your hands to your heart in prayer position and dedicate the merit of your practice to the benefit of all beings. Bow toward your heart and, with care and presence, return to your day.

Almost at the end of our spring season practices, we've journeyed through the four layers of your being — your body, mind, emotions, and spirit — and learned how best to support them at this time of year. Now let's take a step back and reflect on what you've learned, created, given, and received along the way. True growth happens when you pause and reflect on where you've been. Only then can you integrate your lessons to forge a clear path forward. Carve out some quiet time, grab your journal, and let's go...

REMEMBER

- Use the spring yoga and meditation sequences to cultivate the energetic qualities needed for health and harmony this season: creativity, focus, determination, steadiness, and kindness.
- Use yin yoga to gently tone and enliven your liver and gallbladder meridians, especially when suffering from PMS, hot flashes, and mood swings or when feeling run-down, indecisive, shut off from your anger, or agitated.
- Try a vigorous yoga flow to build your body heat, stimulate digestion and lymph, break up winter stagnation, and shed excess weight.
- Practice loving-kindness for yourself as often as you can to cultivate self-love and acceptance. Then move on, and share it with others.

Chapter 9

SPRING REFLECTIONS

The final step in your rebirthing process is to step back and contemplate all you've done. How have these practices affected you? Your family? Your community? The following journaling topics are opportunities for you to see and digest everything you've put into place in your inner and outer life this season. Write about these topics whenever you feel called to or when you have time (in the waiting room at the dentist, on the airplane, before you go to sleep, in the bathtub). Remember, these exercises need more than your mental contemplation. Alchemy happens when you write. Here the deeper wisdom of your soul can shine through, and ultimately that's the place we all want to live from.

I've broken these topics down month by month so you can complete them in bite-size chunks as you go. Feel free to find other creative ways to document your journey: make a collage with pictures of key moments, use finger paints to paint how you feel. At the end of the season, step back and look at your creations all together. You can also collect small items from nature to place on your altar as you go to remind you of your growing connection to the natural world.

MONTH ONE

1. At the start of this season, I felt stuck in the following ways:
2. My main health concerns were:
3. The three main toxic thoughts I have or stories I tell myself regularly are:
4. The physical space that most needs detoxing and decluttering is:
5. The one habit I'm going to really focus on cultivating for the next thirty days is _____. I will omit _____ in order to create space for this. The main things I hope to feel as a result of this are:

MONTH TWO

1. The biggest step I've taken this month to detox my body has been _____, and the results I'm feeling are _____ and _____.
2. When I was a little girl the four ways I most loved to be creative were:
3. This month I have wanted to focus on making more time for the childhood creative act of:
4. I've spent most of my spare time this month:
5. The strong emotions I've experienced most this season are _____ and _____. I think they're trying to tell me that I need to change _____ and _____.

MONTH THREE

1. The three things I'm celebrating most from my efforts this season are:
2. Looking back, I realize my three biggest challenges were:
3. Even though I didn't _____ so well, I still learned a big lesson, which is _____.
4. The five main ways I plan to continue connecting with nature regularly are:
5. The dream I have in my soul that I still want to bring into the world is: By learning how to focus, direct, and apply our creative life force — by

COMMUNITY RITUAL

Find ways to connect with the people you love to honor this season. Invite some friends (or your children's friends) over to paint Easter eggs. Plan a huge Seder dinner. Go to the farmers' market with a girlfriend or family member. Make one of the meals from this chapter and have a dinner party. Join or start a women's circle, and meet on the full and new moon each month. Do the one-day retreat with this circle of friends. Doing so helps to bring your inner world out and lets others know about all the ways you're growing and changing. Listen to how others experienced this season too. To find a women's group near you and to share your experiences, visit www.TheWayoftheHappyWoman.com.

both clearing out the old and bringing in the new, we ready ourselves to delight in the colorful manifestations and the bright fullness of summer. What will summer's warm breezes reveal?

PART 3

SUMMER

Element: FIRE

Color: RED

Organs: HEART AND SMALL INTESTINE

Heart qualities: HATE AND COMPASSION

Life cycle: EARLY ADULTHOOD

Creative cycle: FRUITION

Menstrual cycle: OVULATION AND FERTILITY

Moon cycle: FULL MOON

Actions: PLAYING, REJOICING, AND ENJOYING

Focus: CELEBRATE ALL THAT IS LUSH, FULL,
AND FLOURISHING IN YOUR LIFE.

Chapter 10

REJOICING

Bare feet, watermelon, sunburns, and sipping Chardonnay on the deck under the stars: all reflect summer's freedom, joy, and playfulness. On June 21 in the northern hemisphere (and on December 21 in the southern), the summer solstice burns brightly as the longest day of the year — so bright that in northern lands such as Alaska and Scandinavia, the sun never even sets that evening. From this point onward, the sun's yang energy slowly wanes, as do the daylight hours, until we reach the darkest point in the yearly spectrum, the winter solstice. The impermanence of this bright day signifies the earth's biggest inhalation of the year and reminds us to celebrate and relish all of life's pleasures by drinking them into every cell of our bodies.

Just as a child savors each day of her summer vacation, counting down the days until her return to school, we also must become more present and more attuned to the warmth, colorfulness, fecundity, and juiciness of this season through even the simplest of pleasures. It's time to partake in nature's flourishing and to celebrate all the ways in which our lives are blossoming too.

The ancient Chinese celebrated the earth, the feminine, and the yin forces on summer's arrival. Ancient pagans honored midsummer with bonfires; Swedes decorated a midsummer tree to dance around in a magical ritual intended to bring rain. Caribbean pirates believed a ship could sail off the world and into the sun on that day, and Native Americans have created countless stone structures linked to equinoxes and solstices, the most famous being Wyoming's Bighorn Medicine Wheel.

Make it a priority to enjoy summer's delicacies as you go about your life. Enjoy walks in the morning air, yoga outdoors, lunches in the park, moments to watch the sun rise or set, bike rides through the country, candlelit dinners on the deck, or afternoons spent swimming and sunning at the beach or pool. Even indulging in quick snapshots of summer can do it: sip a fresh juice, sunbathe on the roof during your lunch break, or wear a bright flower in your hair to work.

The season invites us to bring more enthusiasm, warmth, extroversion, and joy into our daily lives, to be as energetic as children. We can stay up late and wake up early, like the sun. We can splash in swimming holes or nap under the shaded canopy of a big tree to escape midafternoon heat. We can bite into a ripe mango or a juicy peach.

THE PLEASURE PRINCIPLE

You alone are responsible for your happiness. You can't count on a relationship, a new job, or a great pair of shoes to supply it. Sure, those things make everything feel rosy for a while, but I'm talking about real, deep-down, heart-felt bliss, when you know that all is well with the world. Living from that place takes a willingness to find it within you. Is your longing to be truly happy strong enough that you're willing to regularly step away from your job, your computer, and your phone? To engage in things that let you live in the present moment and bring you innocent joy and pleasure? Your life's not going to slow down. People are always going to want something from you. If you're not doing something every day that brings you total bliss, you need to ask yourself, "Why not?" Denying yourself delight will lead you down a path of isolation, blame, and an aching neediness as you look for others to fulfill you. Permitting yourself to partake in pleasure is the most important factor in your mental and physical health. You can't be truly healthy or happy without pleasure. It's the catalyst for a series of biochemical reactions in your brain and body — caused primarily by the release of the love hormone, oxytocin — that bring radiance, fluidity, positivity, and an underlying sense of well-being.

The ironic thing is that at a certain level we are all afraid to feel blissful.

TRY THIS

Pour yourself a glass of Cool Mint Tea (recipe on page 154), find a shady spot, and reflect on the following summertime musings in your journal.

Brainstorm concrete ways that you can bring more simple pleasures into your days this summer. What really makes you come alive? What did you love to do as a young girl at this time of year? Come up with at least twenty to thirty ideas — it doesn't matter how simple (or zany) they are!

I'll include a few to get you started:

- Paint your nails bright red.
- Ride a horse.
- Buy some kids' sidewalk chalk, and write inspiring quotes and draw big hearts on the sidewalk.
- Get naked: go skinny-dipping, take a moon bath, or forgo your PJs when you sleep.
- Turn on your sprinkler and run through it.
- Get a chair massage for ten minutes at the farmers' market.

This state involves deep feelings and sensations, which are sometimes as unbearable as pain and suffering. On top of that, we have few role models in the world who revel in their beauty, their bodies, and the ecstasy of being alive. The summer, in her unabashed lushness, can serve as your role model. A rose doesn't keep herself from unfurling because she's afraid her scent will be too overbearing or intoxicating or that her petals will be too soft and ostentatious. Using nature as your teacher, find the courage to bring more pleasure into your world. Ask yourself, "What's holding me back from making pleasure a priority in my life? Am I afraid to feel really good and to let everyone see me this way?"

Renée, a South African living in the Philippines, came to one of my women's yoga workshops in Bangkok with her hair tied back in a ponytail and wearing a baggy tank top and worn yoga pants. She seemed quiet, tired, and a little detached. During one of the morning practices, I had the women hold Chair Pose for what they perceived to be an ungodly length of time (about three minutes, in reality). In the midst of it, nearly all of them stopped breathing and tensed up their faces until I asked them to soften, to feel supported by Mother Earth beneath them, and to breathe even more deeply than they thought possible. Moments later, Renée's whole body started quivering, and tears streamed down her cheeks. A big smile slowly spread across her face as she sank deeper into the pose with newfound strength and clarity. Later on, during one of our sharing circles, she revealed her realization from the morning: she had been managing her busy life (working, raising her family, caring for her aging mother) by controlling everything, even her body. Everything had a strict schedule and a set way to be. She had thought that goofing off for an hour, dressing beautifully, or even taking the time to pick out the perfect pair of earrings each day was too self-indulgent and took too much time. With all her rigid routines to "fit everything in," she had completely lost touch with her own pleasure. When she allowed herself to lose control during that one intense yoga pose, she realized how much stronger she could be if she allowed herself to feel more, shine more, and acknowledge how supported she truly was in that process.

THE FIRE ELEMENT

Part of this season's frivolousness comes from its ruling element: fire. This flickering flame breaks up any residual heaviness from the spring and sheds the sunlight on your life that you need for your creative projects to bloom into maturity. It can only burn from the healthy wood of the spring season — meaning that fruition of dreams only comes from the fuel of intentional creativity.

When it's in balance, this fire gives you a love of life and infuses you with an infectious inner light and motherly warmth. It also inspires you to reach out, communicate well, and get out there to network and make connections. You'll feel inclined to bring your neighbor a few of the cookies you baked last night or to call up a friend in distress and ask her what you can do to support her. Too little fire equals melancholy and a low libido (and sluggish digestion, as you'll find out in the next chapters); too much fire shows up as agitation, restlessness, and a tendency to blow up over minutiae. Generally, it's not acceptable for women to express their anger. If they do they're called "bitches" or "lunatics." Finding non-harming ways to release anger — feeling in your body where this fire lives, then stomping your feet to African drums, screaming into your pillow, or roaring like a lioness in your women's circle — will help you to harness the clarifying fierceness of your fire energy without projecting it onto others unskillfully.

S U M M E R   R E T R E A T

ONE-DAY SUMMER PLEASURE RETREAT

While I urge you to continue with the daily rhythms (outlined on page 26), you can also partake in this one-day retreat to fully incorporate the food, lifestyle, and yoga practices for summer. Remember to unplug today — turn off your phone, and power down your computer! Pay extra attention to your sensuality. Feel the sun and breeze on your skin. Drink in the colors and scents of nature fully. Receive this season's bountiful beauty.

- Get out of bed between 6:00 and 7:00 A.M. to take advantage of the bright morning and cool breezes. Drink a glass or two of water, and brew peppermint or rose tea.
- Sit for ten minutes in Compassion Meditation (page 176).
- Practice the summer flow yoga practice (page 166). If it's warm enough and you have the outdoor space (a rooftop, backyard, or deck), do it there.
- Do some skin brushing (page 83), and massage your whole body with coconut oil (page 190). (You can also massage some coconut oil into your scalp and hair and onto your feet before bed — a beauty secret of Indian women.) Then take a hot shower, followed by a cold water blast.
- Make the summer breakfast smoothie (recipe on page 140).

- Choose some of the reflections from chapter 13, or write three stream-of-consciousness pages in your journal.
- Spend your morning outside: in the botanical gardens, at the park, at the beach; at the farmers' market; blueberry picking, hiking, or window shopping in your favorite neighborhood. Go without any agenda. Inhale the beauty all around you — colors, sights, scents, sounds, tastes.
- Eat lunch in an outdoor café, or get takeout (or bring your own bag lunch) for a picnic.
- Before heading home, be sure to buy yourself (or if you're in the outdoors pick a wildflower bouquet) a little something that you normally wouldn't. It doesn't have to be expensive — a cute headband, magnetic poetry for your refrigerator, some sexy thong underwear, or a new pair of flip-flops.
- Rehydrate at home with a tall glass of regular or cucumber water (recipe on page 157). Refresh yourself with a splash of rose water. *Tip:* To make your own rose water, add one drop of rose oil (from India or Bulgaria) to a gallon of water. Shake it, and take one drop of this mixture and add it to another fresh gallon of water. You can then put this in a spray bottle for a face mist or room spray or sip on it for a refreshing drink.
- Do a walking meditation outside with your bare feet on the grass for ten minutes or more (page 178).
- Enjoy a nap or rest. Play some beautiful, relaxing music. Inhale deeply and receive it.
- Read a book about creativity or sexuality for about an hour, followed by finger painting, sketching, watercoloring, rock painting, knitting, gardening, cooking, or another creative project in which you feel no attachment to the outcome.
- Do the summer yin yoga practice (page 162).
- Invite a friend (or friends) over for dinner. Fire up the grill, or make the Veggie Pesto Pasta (recipe on page 156) — and don't forget the dessert!
- Spend the evening socializing, playing Scrabble, singing karaoke, or doing whatever elicits fun for you.

SUMMER RETREAT

- Before bed, step outside and bathe in the stars and the moon.
- To wind down, rub your feet and scalp with coconut oil. Lie down on your bed and put your legs up the wall as you breathe deeply and reflect on everything you're grateful for from the day.
- Lights out before midnight. (It's summertime, and you usually need less sleep!)

SUMMER MOON TIME PRACTICES

This season's warm temperatures allow for some great moon practices. On the full moon, get naked, wrap yourself in a big blanket, and at night privately slip outside onto your roof or into your backyard. If your house isn't private enough, get together with a girlfriend who has a more secluded space to do this. Lie down on the earth, your back on the blanket. Drink the moonlight into your body. Bathe in it. Pray to the moon for any healing of your body, sexuality, or femininity that you need right now. If there's some water nearby, go for a moonlit skinny-dip.

During your menstrual cycle in the summer (and year-round), use organic cloth menstrual pads (I like www.PartyPantsPads.com; they're much friendlier to the environment and your body than the disposable ones) most of the time and organic tampons when you are going to the beach or want to go swimming. Pads allow the downward flow of your menstrual blood to remain uninterrupted, so they're the best option. I know it might sound a little far-out for many of you, but, ideally, each day you should soak your soiled menstrual pads in a large jar that's filled with cold water. Then, at the end of the day, wash the pads in the washing machine with cold water, and feed your favorite plant or tree the water from the jar. Why on earth would you want to do that, you might ask? Well, menstrual blood hasn't always been seen as dirty or gross. Our ancestors thought menstrual blood to be very rejuvenating and fertilizing, and in ancient times, women sat on the earth in red tents and moon lodges, bleeding directly into the ground beneath them. Some of my women friends involve their daughters in this ritual each month to teach them how to revere, rather than hide, their menstrual blood.

I first learned this when I spent the summer at one of my teacher's ashrams in the Pyrenees of southern France. She mentioned this ancient wisdom, and, since I was camping at the time, I had plenty of opportunities to squat on the earth and release my menstrual blood. Because my mind was so quiet during those months due to a lot of yoga and meditation practices (and living in such

SEX IT UP

Summer's the most fertile season of the year. Similar to a woman's monthly ovulation, summer, with its juicy fruits and sultry breezes, invites you into a sensual dance. To be a healthy woman, you need to cultivate a healthy sex life. However, one of the most wounded parts of a woman's soul is her sexuality. Considering that one out of every three women you know has suffered some sort of sexual abuse in her lifetime, this comes as no surprise. And yet our nature is inherently sexual, for simply being alive in a woman's body is hugely erotic. In fact, our sexuality is one of the most powerful portals into our spirituality, indigenous power, and authentic happiness — but only when we heal our relationship with it and recover this innocent eroticism. Did you know that orgasms actually benefit your health tremendously? They infuse every cell of your being with a cocktail of feel-good hormones. It's no coincidence that after good sex your skin looks dewier and more radiant and your eyes shine!

How can you begin to first heal your relationship with your sexual energy and then cultivate it — so that it becomes part of your self-care, your connection with spirit and your intimate partner, and a path to embodied fullness? Here are a few things to try:

- Take a hot bath filled with pink rose petals. Light candles all around. Rub your body with coconut oil, and step into the tub. Using one of the rose petals, very slowly, attentively, and lightly touch every inch of your body. Feel the sensations, and breathe deeply. Inhale, and hug to you whatever you experience.
- Buy yourself some sexy lingerie. Don't save it for special occasions. If your intimate partner sees it, great. But wear it for *you.* You'll feel sexy in an instant.
- Make self-pleasuring a regular part of your life, even if you're in a relationship. Make regular "sex dates" with yourself to explore your body. Light candles, and turn on music. Don't forget to include foreplay. Learn what truly turns you on, what feels good, and what doesn't feel good.
- Get yourself some books on sexual anatomy, the stages of your arousal, and the different types of orgasms you can have. You can find the ones I recommend on my website.
- Have a sex date with your partner. Let him or her be completely passive so that you have the chance to take things at your own pace — stroking hair, nibbling on an earlobe. Then change roles.
- Take a striptease, tango, belly dancing, or pole dancing class (they're everywhere now!).

intimacy with the elements), I could hear the earth — and my inner wisdom — speaking to me, telling me how much she needed women to remember our bond with her. We don't need to keep our menstrual blood so neat and tidy. Sure, we need to be practical and use some discretion at times, but simply by pouring your menstrual water back onto nature's creations, you're helping to heal a long-lost bond between women and our mother, the earth. Your menstrual blood is purifying and powerful and is never something to be ashamed or afraid of.

CELEBRATE SUMMER!

Here are a few more fun ways to celebrate summer that you can incorporate into your days:

- Keep an eye out for animals and insects. Often they come into our lives to deliver a message. Take note of what you come across, and then research what that could mean for you. Trust synchronicities!
- Stargaze. The Australian Aborigines believe that we need to look at the stars more and bring their magic in through our bodies, down into our feet, and into the earth, which needs the medicine of starlight.
- Go berry picking, or gather flowers for your home.
- Walk barefoot on the grass, soil, or sand as much as you can.
- Meditate on the songs of birds during your morning meditation, journaling, or walk.
- Sit on the porch during a thunderstorm and smell the rain.
- Take your art projects outside: paint rocks, watercolor, finger paint.
- Go camping (even if it's just sleeping in your backyard for a night).
- Ride your bike or walk more instead of driving.
- Spend time near water — kayak, canoe, swim, or sail.
- Even when you're working inside, get at least twenty minutes of direct sunlight a day.

THE LATE-SUMMER SEASON

We all feel the distinct shift that happens toward the end of summer, when children head back to school, when it's time to face the piles of work on our desks, and when the setting sun hints of autumn's arrival. The late-summer season, from mid-August until the fall equinox on September 22, holds aspects of all the seasons, for the days can feel sticky and hot or suddenly cool and crisp.

Now the dominant element is earth — or the ash produced from the fire. The organ focus shifts from the heart and small intestine to the stomach, spleen, and pancreas. Late summer's color is yellow (think peaches and summer squashes), and the dominant taste is sweet. While you're winding down from all the summer festivities, now's an important time to stay grounded and to pay special attention to eating well (especially by avoiding too many sugar-laden sweets), for your immunity's more vulnerable from now through the fall. Doing so will help keep you healthy as the colder months of autumn and winter approach.

Emotionally, this transition can be difficult. It's hard to let go of the long days and the levity of spirit that summer gives us. One reason we find this time of year so precious is that we know it won't last forever. Kim, a student in Boulder, helped me to remember this lesson during a women's yoga class she attended. It was her first time at one of these classes, and we were in the process of checking in with one another.

It came time for Kim to speak. Sitting cross-legged and dressed in a cropped T-shirt to show off her toned belly, she nervously twirled a strand of her sun-bleached hair between her fingers. She stared at the wood floor. After several moments of pregnant silence, tears began to pour down her face.

"I'm so scared for summer to end," she said, voice quivering.

The rest of us breathed deeply, as if to drink in a breath for her. "My heart and soul are in the summertime. I love being outside, going to the pool with my kids, being in the garden," she continued, still staring at the floor. "You know, I'm not from here. I'm not a winter person. I get so cold. I don't know what to do with myself when everything dies and everyone goes inside."

An avid cyclist and former surfer, Kim was used to being very active. In fact, she embodied the very medicine that I needed in my early twenties: the vigor and enthusiasm to temporarily suspend obligations and to just get out and enjoy life. In turn, I had just the medicine she craved. She learned how to relax during *savasana* (the final resting pose in yoga) without fidgeting. She started to add contemplative and cooling forward bends and inversions to her active regime. She even took an interest in meditation.

Kim knew, with a childlike passion, how to enjoy summertime, yet she was clinging to it too tightly. The first frost of autumn had the power to erase her joy and strip away her life force. Summer entices us not only to delight in her sweetness but also to remember that this is only one of life's many flavors. The flowers that we cut and place in vases on our dining room tables remind us to celebrate both the flourishing and the inevitable passing of life itself. In this knowing rests the possibility to experience — and live from — true happiness.

REMEMBER

- Carve out more opportunities to bring playfulness, fun, and celebration into your life. Throw a party (or wear more flirty sundresses), go skinny-dipping with your sweetie once the kids go to sleep, or buy yourself some sand toys and build a sand castle instead of reading that gossip magazine.
- Reflect on what makes you happy and lights you up. Figure out the last time you did those things. What can you commit to experiencing again as a regular part of your life?
- Find ways to keep cool: exercise in the morning, massage yourself with coconut oil, make a rosewater face spray to mist yourself and your surroundings during the hottest parts of the day.

Chapter 11

IN *the* KITCHEN
Colorful Celebrations

I have a thing for rainbows. They're a girlhood fascination I'll never outgrow. Who doesn't think it's her lucky day when she sees a rainbow after a summer storm? Following the cool reprieve of booming afternoon thunderstorms, they arc across the sky, adding a splash of bright color, and, on seeing them, we're reminded: yes, magic does exist.

We find summer's colorful display everywhere at this time of year: in the sky, on neon-striped beach towels, within our gardens, and in the medley of fruit on our kitchen counters. Just as a bright, tender tomato calls you to eat it at just the right moment — when it's neither too ripe nor too sour — this season calls you to play with her, delight in her, before she passes. One practical way to do this daily is through the foods that we prepare, share, and eat.

EAT A RAINBOW EVERY DAY

Year-round, one way to ensure that we're sated by the foods we eat and that we're getting a wide range of nutrients and flavors is through making a rainbow on our plate.

In his television series *Food Revolution*, Jamie Oliver offered a great visual demonstration of this. On one show, he went into the home of one American family and emptied their freezer and refrigerator and laid everything out, unwrapped, on the kitchen table for the family to see. Brown, yellow, and white: these were the colors of the potato chips, frozen chicken nuggets, pizzas, bread, and breakfast pastries. No greens. No reds. No blues. No rainbow there. If you want to avoid falling into the dullness of the standard American diet, opt for dynamic color at every meal to ensure your taste buds — and your vitamin and mineral reserves — find harmonic pleasure. Shred a beet (red) in a green salad.

Add toasted sunflower seeds (white) and yellow cherry tomatoes. Sprinkle some dulse flakes (purple) on top, and then serve it all with some steamed sweet potato (orange) on the side.

Many of my coaching clients tell me how summer's the easiest time for them to cut junk food out of their diets. Natural sugars, which are in abundance now, fill the void: nectarines, strawberries, cherries, you name it! It's easy to pick up something healthy and snack on it. Fresh produce floods summertime farmers' markets and roadside stands. Plus, the fire from this season's bright sun and heat induce a natural craving to be satiated by the fresh, watery ingredients that surround us now.

WHAT'S UP WITH RAW FOODS?

One popular nutritional trend is the raw foods diet. As I've mentioned, I'm not a fan of following any set dietary rules and instead encourage you to ask your body what she wants and how much she wants of it — always. Different approaches work at different times, based on what's happening in our bodies and in nature around us.

Having said that, because of summer's heat, and the abundance of fresh produce, the cooling, hydrating qualities of raw foods do make a lot of sense this season. Plus, eating raw does offer many nutritional advantages. Raw foods are still alive — meaning that their enzymes are active because they have not been denatured through cooking (this happens when you cook anything at a temperature above 114°F). You body needs these active enzymes to help initiate its chemical reactions. Since all your body's vital functions rely on these enzymes, many chronic illnesses demonstrate a pronounced decrease in their activity.

That's why many who suffer from terminal illness have gone on supervised raw foods diets, with incredible results. Imbibing the vitality of living foods has restored their life force and thoroughly cleansed their systems. On the flip side, some people, myself included, at times find raw foods hard to digest and too cooling most of the time, especially when eaten in large doses. However, the summer's the perfect time to tap into the healing power of live foods because usually they're what you're craving anyway on a hot day. You'd rather whip up a salad of fresh garden greens for lunch than stand in front of a hot stove stirring up a spicy stew, right? I'll share with you some great raw recipes in the summer menu that follows.

GET JUICY

A great way to incorporate more raw foods into your diet is by juicing. We all know the importance of eating more fruits and vegetables — and that the more you eat the more benefits you reap. However, it's not always easy or practical to eat a big mound of greens every day. When you juice your vegetables, though, you can imbibe massive amounts of these goodies in a single glass. Juicing removes the indigestible fiber from fruits and vegetables and keeps their live enzymes intact.

One easy way to enjoy fresh juice is by drinking the water of young coconuts (the water is clear and very different from the milk, which comes from more mature coconuts). While living in Thailand, I drank a minimum of two coconuts a day — often pulling my motorbike off to the side of the road to buy one icy cold from a nearby stand — to combat the heat and resulting thirst. Way better than any sports drink (with less sugar, less sodium, and more potassium), young coconuts (usually light green or white, not dark brown) are natural isotonic beverages, with the same electrolytic balance that we have in our blood and with the lauric acid that's also present in mother's milk. It has even been used during wartime to give emergency plasma transfusions to wounded soldiers! Now many health food stores around the world sell coconut water in boxes and cans. If you go this route, be sure to buy the unsweetened ones.

SUMMER SHOPPING LIST

Let's make sure that your kitchen is fully stocked now with foods that cool your system, offering the perfect antidote to summer's heat and bringing balance to the fire element.

apricots	carrots
artichokes	cauliflower
asparagus	chard
avocados	cherries
basil	chives
beets	coconuts
berries (all varieties)	collards
broccoli	corn
brown basmati rice	cucumbers
cabbage	eggplant

fava beans	papaya
fennel	parsley
fingerling potatoes	peaches
garlic	peas
green beans	pineapple
lemons	quinoa
lettuce	spinach
mango	sunflower seeds
melons	tomatoes (fresh and sun-dried)
millet	watercress
mint	whole-grain noodles and pastas
mustard greens	(soba, rice, and quinoa)
onion	zucchini/summer squashes

YOUR SUMMER MENU

Here's a full day's worth of recipes to combine summer's bounty in balanced, delicious, and creatively simple ways. Since food carries the intelligence of time and place in its cells, eating local, in-season foods supplies you with the information your body needs to synchronize with summer's spritely rhythm.

BREAKFAST MENU

- Tropical Green Smoothie
- Granola with Almond Milk

TROPICAL GREEN SMOOTHIE

Serves 2

The combination of sweet and savory makes this smoothie a party for your taste buds. Coconut milk adds a lovely richness. Despite the bad rap that coconuts have gotten in the past for being fattening, coconut milk has actually been proven to be fat burning. You can include a low-fat version in smoothies, soups, and salad dressings (the low-fat version is plenty rich and has fewer calories). You can even use it as a dairy substitute in your coffee.

½ small pineapple
1 handful strawberries
½ cup low-fat coconut milk
½ cup water, plus more water or ice as needed
1 scoop brown rice protein powder
½ head romaine lettuce or other lettuce
1 handful cilantro or parsley
4 drops stevia or 1 spoonful raw honey
optional: any superfoods that you enjoy (page 95)

Put pineapple, strawberries, coconut milk, and ½ cup water in a blender, and blend well. Add protein powder, lettuce, cilantro, stevia, and any other superfoods that you'd like. Continue to blend until smooth. Throughout, make sure to add enough water so that all the ingredients are covered.

GRANOLA

Serves 12

This is great for kids and adults as a snack, a tasty breakfast, or a treat while traveling. Serve it with nut milk, low-fat coconut milk, or yogurt, or serve it as a dessert over ice cream or sorbet. You can also just eat it plain by the handful!

3 cups rolled oats
filtered water
1 cup almonds
1 cup sunflower seeds
1 cup pumpkin seeds
½ cup raisins
6 to 7 dates
1 tablespoon vanilla extract
½ teaspoon cinnamon
8 tablespoons raw agave nectar or raw honey
1 teaspoon sea salt

Place rolled oats in 6 cups water, and soak overnight. Place nuts and seeds in a large bowl, cover with water, and soak overnight. Place raisins in a separate bowl, cover with water, and soak overnight. In the morning, place dates in water, and soak for 20 to 30 minutes. Drain and rinse the oats, nuts, seeds, raisins, and dates. (You can water your plants with the soaking water.) Chop the dates into small pieces, removing the pits. In a large bowl, combine oats, nuts, seeds, raisins, and dates. Then add vanilla, cinnamon, agave, and sea salt. Mix together well with your hands. Transfer mixture onto two large parchment-lined baking sheets. Bake the granola in the oven on the lowest setting (usually 135°F) for 24 hours, or use a dehydrator. For a cooked version, bake 1 hour in the oven at 350°F. Serve with fruit and/or fresh almond milk (see recipe below). Store the granola in a sealed glass jar or container, and it will keep for about a month in the refrigerator.

ALMOND MILK

Serves 2

Almonds are very alkaline: they help to neutralize excess acids in the stomach and offer a great supply of high-quality protein and calcium. Plus, this almond milk tastes so much better than what you can buy in cartons at the store!

1 cup raw almonds
3 cups water, plus water for soaking

Soak almonds overnight in water. In the morning, drain and then rinse almonds. Place almonds and 3 cups water in a blender, and blend until the liquid is a creamy white. Strain the milk through a nut-milk bag, cheesecloth, or mesh paint bag (you can purchase one from a hardware store). Discard the almond rinds that remain in the bag, or use them to make Bliss Balls (recipe on page 154). Refrigerate in a sealed container, and use within 3 to 5 days.

TIP: You can also use this almond milk in smoothies. For different flavors, try adding vanilla extract, carob, and a little bit of raw honey or agave (for "chocolate milk"), or some rose water (recipe on page 139).

MORE BREAKFAST IDEAS

- A big bowl of fresh fruit with a handful of soaked nuts and a dash of light coconut milk or coconut milk yogurt and a spoonful of raw, local honey.
- Chia Seed Porridge (recipe on page 253).
- Rice cakes lightly toasted and spread with almond butter.

THE SCOOP ON SWEETENERS

Regular white sugar (and its variants, such as corn syrup) and artificial sweeteners weaken your life force. Here's the lowdown on four of the best sweeteners to use:

1. *Raw, local honey:* Consuming raw, local honey has long been viewed as a way to boost one's immunity (and to help with clearing up pollen allergies). However, for those who are hyperglycemic, honey's not always your best bet. Containing up to 60 percent more sugar than white sugar (and a whole lot more nutrients as well), it's absorbed rapidly into the bloodstream. Also, honey's beneficial enzymes become denatured when heated above 105 degrees. Ayurveda observes that it actually becomes a toxin in the body then, leading to the formation of excess mucus. When I'm cooking (or adding sweetener to a hot tea), I use agave instead. Save honey for sweetening cool drinks or for drizzling on top of your food.

2. *Raw agave nectar:* While agave nectar has received a bad rap recently for not being as hyperglycemic as originally supposed, in my opinion it's still a great sugar alternative, especially for baking and for using in hot beverages. The Aztecs praised it as a gift from the gods and used it to flavor foods and drinks. Produced from southern Mexico's blue agave plant (yup, the same one that tequila comes from), agave tastes and looks much like honey.

3. *Stevia:* A noncaloric herb that's native to Paraguay, stevia has been used as a sweetener and flavor enhancer for centuries and has recently come into style. It is actually sweeter than sugar. You can buy it in white-powder, green-leaf, or clear-extract form. I like to use the extract, adding a few drops to my tea or smoothies.

4. *Xylitol:* Found naturally in berries, fruits, vegetables, and mushrooms, xylitol's Finnish name is *koivusokeri*, or "birch sugar," for the best way to make it comes from chopping up xylan, the structural fiber of the wood. Chemically xylitol is not a sugar, but a sugar alcohol, and it is structurally different from other sweeteners. As a result, most bacteria found in the mouth can't use this form of sugar, making it a potent supplement for dental health. Xylitol chewing gum, mints, and toothpaste have become very popular. You can buy xylitol in a powder and use it as you would white sugar.

LUNCH MENU

- Lavender Lemonade
- Veggie Nori Burritos

LAVENDER LEMONADE

Serves 4

This refreshing tonic won't sap your energy during the midafternoon heat. For a more festive version, use sparkling, rather than spring, water.

 ¼ cup dried lavender
 2 cups boiling water
 ¼ cup agave nectar
 8 lemons
 5 cups cool water
 a few lemon slices for garnish, if you'd like

Place the lavender in a bowl, and pour the boiling water over it. Steep for 10 minutes. Strain out the lavender and discard it. Mix the agave into the hot lavender water. Juice the lemons in a pitcher, and add the cool water and hot lavender water. Refrigerate for about an hour, or serve right away over ice.

VEGGIE NORI BURRITOS

Serves 2

These burritos are great for a picnic or long road trip. Nori is the kind of seaweed used to wrap sushi and is packed with vitamins and minerals. When toasted, it adds a rich, salty, savory accent to any meal. These are fun for kids to make too.

 1 to 2 tablespoons tahini
 2 sheets toasted nori
 1 cup cooked brown rice
 1 avocado, sliced
 1 medium tomato
 6 to 8 large romaine lettuce or spinach leaves, sliced into thin strips
 a handful sunflower sprouts
 1 to 2 tablespoons olive oil
 2 pinches of sea salt

Spread a thin layer of tahini onto each nori sheet. Place half the rice in the center of each sheet. Add the avocado, tomato, greens, and sprouts on top of the rice. Drizzle with olive oil and sprinkle with sea salt. Roll the nori into a cone shape by wrapping the ends around the filling. Seal the end by licking your finger to dampen the edge and create a seal.

TIP: Feel free to improvise. You can wrap so many different things in nori once you get the hang of it.

MORE LUNCH IDEAS

- Wrap all the above ingredients in a brown rice tortilla, replacing the tahini with hummus.
- Leftover roasted veggies with a big, green salad with walnuts, tofu, or your favorite lean protein.
- Soba noodles tossed with raw snap peas and scallions and dressed in tahini and lemon juice.

PRESERVE THE SUMMER

My older sister and I have a tradition of making jam at our summer home on Lake Michigan using fresh local raspberries, blueberries, or strawberries. It's easy and is a great activity to do with your children or girlfriends. Once your jam is made, you can savor summer's bright goodies year-round, and you can also give your jars of jam as gifts. You can freeze berries or other fruits to use in smoothies or pies later, or make fruit leather in a dehydrator.

Here's my favorite fruit jam recipe:

Pick your berries of choice, or buy them freshly picked. If all else fails, frozen works too. You'll need 8 to 10 cups to make one batch. Wash them, remove the stems, and mush them up. You will need a case of mason jars with lids and rings. Sanitize the jars in the dishwasher. Keep them in there (so they stay hot) until you're ready to use them. Stir the berries and a sugar-free pectin (this you can buy at most grocery stores; follow the directions on the box) together in a large pot on medium to high heat. Stir regularly to avoid burning. Bring to a boil. Put the lids in a pan of hot water to soften the gummed surface and make sealing easier. Add 2 cups of apple juice concentrate to the berry/pectin mix, and bring back to a full, hard boil for 1 minute.

Fill jars within ¼ inch of the top, wiping off any spills on the edges. Place the lids on and tighten the rings around them. Put the jars in a big pot of boiling water deep enough that the water reaches two inches above the jar tops, and let them boil in the water for 5 minutes. Lift the jars out of the water and let them cool overnight. Check the seal on the lids. If the lid pops it didn't seal correctly. You can still use this jam, but refrigerate it and eat it right away. The sealed jars can be stored, unrefrigerated, for up to 18 months.

SNACK MENU

- Cool Mint Tea
- Bliss Balls

COOL MINT TEA

Serves 4 to 6

This lovely tea aids digestion and soothes the nerves on a hot day. It's also a great midafternoon refresher.

> 1 quart boiling water
> 1 cup fresh peppermint leaves or ¼ cup dried peppermint
> 2 tablespoons agave nectar
> 1 quart room-temperature water

Pour the boiling water over the peppermint leaves in a teapot or other heat-proof container (I recommend using a big glass mason jar; do not use plastic). Cover and let steep for 20 minutes. Strain tea into a glass pitcher or another mason jar, and stir in agave. Add the cool water. Chill in the refrigerator for at least an hour. Serve with or without ice cubes.

TIP: For a quick, refreshing minty drink, add a drop or two of peppermint oil and lemon oil to water. Make sure you put these in a stainless-steel container (such as water bottle or pitcher), since the lemon will eat away at any other surface. Be sure to use therapeutic-grade essential oils for this, since these are the only ones meant for consumption. I recommend getting them from the Ananda apothecary (www.anandaapothecary.com).

BLISS BALLS

Makes 24 balls

These have earned their name. They're a sweet and energizing treat and are also great to travel with. Plus, they always get rave reviews at parties. I can't even begin to count how many times I have shared this recipe with others. There are endless variations, and you really can't get it wrong. These taste good, no matter what!

2 cups any combination of cashew nuts, almonds, sunflower seeds, pecans, sesame seeds, and/or walnuts (when I have leftover almond pulp from making almond milk I use that)

½ cup carob or unsweetened cocoa powder, plus extra for dusting

1 teaspoon cinnamon

½ teaspoon sea salt

½ cup raisins

½ cup dates, soaked for 20 minutes and then pitted

½ cup almond butter or tahini

2 tablespoons honey or agave nectar

1 teaspoon vanilla extract

optional: 1 teaspoon spirulina or raw coconut flakes.

Put nuts and seeds, carob or cocoa, cinnamon, salt, raisins, and dates in a food processor, and pulse until blended. Add almond butter or tahini, honey or agave, and vanilla and blend until you get a sticky goo. Shape the mixture into ½-inch balls. Dust them with carob or cocoa powder, or roll them in spirulina or coconut flakes. Store them in the refrigerator or freezer.

FROZEN SUMMER TREATS

Freeze grapes or blueberries for a quick, refreshing treat (or dessert). Wash the grapes or berries, let them dry, and then store them in a freezer bag. Grab a handful whenever you want a cooling, sweet snack. Warning: these can be a little addictive because they're so good!

DINNER MENU

- Veggie Pesto Pasta
- Farmers' Market Salad
- My Favorite Salad Dressing
- Cucumber Water

VEGGIE PESTO PASTA

Serves 4

If you make an extra-big batch of these roasted or grilled veggies, you can eat them for a few days on your salads too. You may also want to make a double batch of the pesto and freeze the extra for later — it's great as a dip for veggies or as a sandwich spread.

1 cup sun-dried tomatoes
4 cups vegetables — 3 or 4 different kinds (try summer squash, zucchini, red or yellow bell peppers, or portabella mushrooms)
2 tablespoons, plus ¼ cup olive oil
sea salt and black pepper to taste
1 package brown rice spaghetti
1 cup Italian parsley
1 cup fresh basil leaves
2 small garlic cloves
½ cup raw cashews
½ teaspoon sea salt

Preheat oven to 400°F. In a medium bowl, cover the sun-dried tomatoes with water. Julienne the 4 cups veggies, place them in a large baking dish, and toss well with the 2 tablespoons olive oil and salt and pepper to taste. Bake for about 30 minutes, stirring after 15 minutes. (Alternatively, you could grill the veggies until tender.) While the veggies are in the oven, cook the spaghetti according to the instructions on the package, timing the cooking to coincide with the completion of the veggies. While the veggies and spaghetti are cooking, drain and thinly slice the sun-dried tomatoes. Then, to make the pesto, put the parsley, basil, garlic, cashews, ½ teaspoon salt, and ¼ cup olive oil in a food processor or blender and puree. Rinse and drain the spaghetti and toss with the pesto and tomatoes. Place the veggies on top.

OPTION: Garnish with some fresh basil leaves and crumbled goat cheese or soft tofu.

FARMERS' MARKET SALAD

Serves 4

You can use any sort of fresh greens here. See what looks good to you at your farmers' market, and create away!

 1 small head leafy green lettuce, washed, dried, and torn into bite-size pieces
 ½ bunch watercress, stems discarded, leaves torn into bite-size pieces
 ½ bunch arugula, stems discarded, leaves torn into bite-size pieces
 My Favorite Salad Dressing (recipe follows)

Combine all the greens in a large serving bowl with My Favorite Salad Dressing (see below).

OPTION: For more protein, add 1 cup pecans, walnuts, chickpeas, or edamame (out of the pod).

MY FAVORITE SALAD DRESSING

After my older sister had her first baby I went to stay with her for a few weeks and made most of the meals. One of her favorite items was my salad dressing. When I make it for dinner parties, people always ask for the recipe — yet more evidence that simple's always better!

 2 tablespoons olive oil
 1 tablespoon tamari
 1 tablespoon lemon juice, apple cider vinegar, or balsamic vinegar

Drizzle the olive oil, tamari, and lemon juice or vinegar over the salad. Toss well, and make sure all the leaves are saturated. If you need more liquid, taste first to see if you need more depth (add more oil), bite (add more lemon juice or vinegar), or savoriness (add more tamari).

CUCUMBER WATER

Serves 4 to 6

This is so refreshing and simple, I often make one pitcher a day and leave it sitting on my kitchen counter to sip on throughout the day. The water-packed cucumber eases swelling (put thin slices on your eyes when you're relaxing or soaking in the tub for a mini-facial). A pitcher of this water also looks quite elegant on the dinner table.

½ organic cucumber, thinly sliced
2 quarts spring or filtered water

Place the cucumber in a large glass pitcher or mason jar. Add water, and let sit for several hours. Serve chilled or at room temperature, depending on your preference.

MORE DINNER IDEAS

- Gazpacho with quinoa and a Farmers' Market Salad.
- A gluten-free pizza crust (try Bob's Red Mill) with tomato or pesto sauce, baby spinach, roasted tomatoes, and fennel. Add a little goat cheese or soft tofu, if you'd like.
- Thai green curry (with light coconut milk and Thai Kitchen's green curry paste) with carrots, broccoli, and your protein of choice. Serve with brown basmati rice.

DESSERT MENU

- Chocolate Avocado Mousse

CHOCOLATE AVOCADO MOUSSE

Serves 4

Both children and adults love this one. It's nothing but rich, smooth, creamy, and chocolatey goodness — without the processed sugars that would normally leave you feeling sleepy after a big meal.

4 avocados
1 cup unsweetened cocoa
1 cup agave nectar
1 tablespoon vanilla extract

Blend all ingredients in a food processor or blender until creamy. Serve chilled.

OPTION: Add a bit of rosewater (recipe on page 139) and/or garnish with a sprig of fresh mint or fresh berries.

TIP: One of my favorite store-bought summer frozen desserts is Coconut Bliss "ice cream" (especially the Mint Galactica and Cherry Amaretto). Made with coconut milk and agave instead of milk and white sugar, it's not only delicious but also very healthy.

Remember, these recipes are not meant to be just another thing to add to your voluminous to-do list. Even if you choose just one, make it with full attention and care. My summer staple is a big salad of fresh produce from the farmers' market tossed with My Favorite Dressing. I might add some avocado, garbanzo beans, grilled salmon, or quinoa or millet on the side. Be casual and creative, but most of all, enjoy yourself.

Now that you're well nourished, grab a glass of your cucumber water, and let's step onto the yoga mat.

REMEMBER

- Indulge in the colors of the season: make a rainbow on your plate!
- Favor fresh fruits and vegetables. Raw foods will keep you cool and hydrated during this fiery season.
- Capture the summer's magic year-round by freezing or dehydrating fruit or by making preserves.
- Find ways to connect with others in festive ways during mealtimes: eat outdoors, go on picnics, have friends over for a barbeque.

Chapter 12

ON *the* YOGA MAT
In Full Bloom

Just as watermelon cools us off and quenches our thirst on sultry summer afternoons, our yoga postures can do the same. At this time of the year you want to choose a yoga routine that will cool you down, calm fiery emotions such as agitation or overambition, and connect you with joy, celebration, and playfulness.

During the summer, it's best to practice in the early-morning or evening hours, when the sun's intensity has subsided a bit. I love unrolling my yoga mat outdoors whenever possible — on the patio, deck, lawn, or rooftop — to really participate in the beauty of the season. It's also a great time to practice with friends: make a date to do partner yoga in the park under the shade of big trees. Use the heat to light your inner creative spark while limbering up and lengthening tight muscles; let it help you explore new depths in your postures. If a home yoga practice isn't for you, go for a jog on the beach, a hike, or a long bike ride.

EMOTIONAL AND MENTAL QUALITIES
OF THE HEART AND SMALL INTESTINE

The summer yin yoga sequence targets the heart and the small intestine, which, although physically distant from each other in the body, work closely together to govern the body's blood flow, in both the physical and energetic senses, since blood is considered an aspect of your life force, or chi. As everyone who has ever suffered from a broken heart knows, your heart plays a prominent role in helping you feel alive, vibrant, and connected. When it's healthy you feel warm, nourished, and able to build healthy relationships. When it's out of balance, you may feel disconnected, depressed, or isolated. Conversely, you could feel hyperactive, agitated, and quick-tempered — common for many of us when we have too many irons in the fire.

Healthy qualities of the small intestine chi include experiencing clear emotions and sorting through things. Together, these qualities connect us to our source of innate happiness, regardless of what's happening in our external environment.

EMOTIONAL QUALITIES
OF THE SPLEEN AND STOMACH MERIDIANS

More activated in the late summer, the spleen and stomach work closely with digestion and are most affected by our diet. The spleen performs a crucial function: it extracts the nutritional essences from the foods we eat and transforms them into our chi and blood. If our spleen chi is out of balance, we can feel dull, anxious, inflexible, ungrounded, and low on energy, and our biological rhythms, related to sleeping, eating, and thinking, can be disrupted. When it is balanced, we feel cyclical harmony — at home on this earth, in our bodies, in our senses, and in ourselves.

THE LEFT AND THE RIGHT OF IT

Each season we'll be alternating the dominant leg and side in our yoga practice. Usually we do poses on the right side first, but it's good to practice going both ways. In many ancient traditions the left side of the body governs the feminine principle, and the right side governs the masculine. Because of this, it's nice to honor both sides equally. Last season we started everything on the right side, so this season we'll begin on the left.

SUMMER YIN YOGA

This practice stimulates the heart and small intestine meridians, both of which are housed in the upper body, as well as the late-summer organ pair of the stomach and spleen. The heart meridian consists of three branches that grow out of the heart, the first of which passes through the diaphragm and into the small intestine. The second travels up the throat, through the tongue, and to the eye; and the third runs across the chest and along the line of the underside of the arm to the little finger.

The small intestine meridian mirrors the heart meridian by starting at the little finger and running up the topside of the arm to the shoulder. Here it bisects, and one branch descends into the heart, diaphragm, and stomach. The second branch journeys up to the eye and ear. The following yin poses gently stretch and compress these energy lines.

Starting on the inside of the big toe, the spleen meridian travels up the inner leg, just next to the liver meridian. It enters the torso through the groin and passes through the stomach and spleen, then ascends through the chest and heart and terminates at the back of the tongue. Its complement, the stomach meridian, starts to the side of the nose and travels through the diaphragm, stomach, and spleen. It travels down the top of the leg and ends at the second toe.

Before Beginning: Review the sections "Create a Sacred Space" (page 67) and "Yin Yoga" (page 49).

Intention: To cool and calm the body, mind, and emotions and to create a sense of inner nourishment and well-being.

Total Practice Time: 60 minutes

Full Sequence of Illustrations: Below

SUMMER YIN YOGA SEQUENCE

1. Check-In and Intention

2. Cooling Breath

3. Butterfly Pose

4. Sphinx Pose

5. Sphinx or Seal Pose

6. Dragon Pose

7. Wide-Knee Child's Pose with Twist

8. Lateral Dragonfly Pose

9. Full Forward Fold

10. Final Relaxation

11. Compassion Meditation

12. Dedication of Merit

1. *Check-In and Intention* (2 to 3 minutes): You can review these in chapter 3.
2. *Cooling Breath* (1 to 2 minutes): Bring your attention to your natural breath, letting it linger on the exhalation. Follow your breath all the way to the end. As you inhale, imagine that you're breathing in cool air, and as you exhale, imagine that you're breathing out excess heat. Use this same breath concentration throughout the practice to cool and quiet your system.
3. *Butterfly Pose* (5 minutes): Uncross your legs and bring the soles of your feet together so they touch, creating a wide diamond shape in the negative space inside your legs. Stay sitting upright, or bend forward over your legs to create an even arch through your front and back spine. If it feels okay for your neck, dangle your head, or rest it in your palms or on a cushion. To come out, unfurl slowly and stretch out your legs. Now come down to lie on your belly.

4. *Sphinx Pose* (5 minutes): See page 110.
5. *Seal* or *Sphinx Pose* again (5 minutes): See page 110. Press back into Child's Pose by placing your hands under your shoulders and inhaling up onto your hands and knees, and exhaling as you take your hips back to rest on your heels, big toes touching, arms stretched out overhead. Rest here for 3 to 5 breaths. Then lift your hips up and come onto your hands and knees.

6. *Dragon Pose* (5 minutes on each side): Step your left foot forward between your hands, keeping your right knee on the ground behind you. Inhale and lift up your torso, resting your hands on your front thigh. If this feels like too much of a stretch on your back thigh, bow forward, and place one hand on a block on either side of your front foot. Lunge your hips as far forward and down as feels manageable. Keep your front heel on the ground. After 5 minutes, come back onto your hands and knees, then Child's Pose, and then repeat on the right side.

7. *Wide-Knee Child's Pose with Twist* (5 minutes on each side): From Child's Pose, take your thighs as far apart as they can go, keeping your big toes touching. Inhale and prop yourself up on your forearms, and exhale as you lace your left arm underneath your right underarm, so your left cheek and shoulder come to the ground. On your next inhalation, reach your right

arm back behind you and take hold of the waistline of your pants or hold on to the top of your left thigh with your right hand. Roll the front of your right shoulder away from the floor. Repeat on the other side.

    To come out, bring your knees back together into Child's Pose, then press up to a seated position, swing your hips to one side, and open your legs out wide.

8. *Lateral Dragonfly Pose* (5 minutes on each side): With your legs wide open, bring your left elbow down to the floor in front of your left knee. Prop it up on a block or blanket if you need more height. Rest the left side of your face in your left palm, and stretch your right arm alongside your right ear. Keep both sides of your waist long, your left ribs rolling up toward the ceiling. Repeat on the other side.

    To come out, grip your thighs with your hands and draw your legs back together. *Note:* For cases of sciatica or hamstring injuries, please bend your knees.

9. *Full Forward Fold* (5 minutes): With your legs together, inhale and lengthen your spine, and on the exhale fold forward over your legs. Elongate your arms next to your shins, and rest your head on a cushion or two (placed on your shins) if you need to. Keep the front of your body long and the spinal curve even. To come out, inhale and slowly rise.

10. *Final Relaxation* (5 to 10 minutes): See page 126.

11. *Compassion Meditation* (5 to 10 minutes): Cross your legs (the other leg on top now), and follow the meditation instructions on page 177.

12. *Dedication of Merit* (1 minute): Please revisit this on page 52.

MINI-SUMMER YIN PRACTICE

Short on time? String these three poses together for a fifteen-minute practice. Try them during your lunch break, as your child naps, before your morning shower, or just before sleep.

1. Butterfly Pose
2. Sphinx or Seal Pose
3. Full Forward Fold

SUMMER FLOW YOGA

This practice complements the yin sequence. After having cooled and quieted your system, now you can flow through some more dynamic shapes. Keep it slow, though, so you don't build excessive heat and leave yourself feeling agitated. Let the exuberance of the postures fill you with an inner glow that shines out to everyone around you, while you stay centered and grounded. Throughout the movements, concentrate on your inhalation as a practice in receiving more. Let this be a dance in which you delight in your own delicious fullness. This practice is also a nice pick-me-up for days when you're feeling lonely or struck with the "mean reds" (as Audrey Hepburn as Holly Golightly so aptly renamed the blues), since it gently enlivens the heart.

Before Beginning: Review the sections "Create a Sacred Space" (page 67) and "Yang (or Flow) Yoga" (page 50).

Intention: To cultivate a cool, quieting tempo while generating feelings of celebration, joy, connection, and shining from the inside out, as the summer sun does.

Total Practice Time: 60 minutes

Full Sequence of Illustrations: Pages 167–69

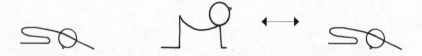

1. *Check-In and Intention* (2 to 5 minutes): Please revisit chapter 3 for details.
2. *Child's Pose with Three-Part Breathing* (3 minutes): Come to Child's Pose with your knees slightly apart so that your belly rests between your inner thighs. Stretch your arms out on the mat in front of you. As you inhale, first fill your lower belly and womb, then let your breath fill your belly and your solar plexus, and finish the inhale by filling up your heart, neck, and head. Then exhale fully, emptying out from the heart and solar plexus, and draw your belly up and back toward your spine. Let your breath move like a wave, through all three of these parts. Close your eyes and really feel the breath moving. Notice what feels good as you breathe, and appreciate that. You'll continue this three-part breath throughout the practice.
3. *Cow Pose* to *Child's Pose Flow:* Inhale and come up onto your hands and knees. Pause here and exhale. As you inhale, using the three-part breath,

SUMMER FLOW YOGA SEQUENCE

1. Check-In and Intention

2. Child's Pose with Three-Part Breathing

3. Cow Pose

Child's Pose

4. Lion's Roar

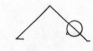

5. Downward-Facing Dog

6. Three-Legged Dog

7. Deep Lunge

8. Downward-Facing Dog

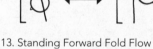

9. Three-Legged Dog with Bent Leg

10. Pigeon Pose

11. Pigeon Pose Thigh Stretch

12. Downward-Facing Dog

13. Standing Forward Fold Flow

14. Standing Forward Fold

15. Mountain Pose

16. Moon Salutations *(3 rounds each side)*

Raised-Arm Mountain Pose

Standing Forward Fold Flow

Low Lunge

Downward-Facing Dog

Plank Pose

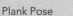

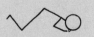

Modified Push-Up

SUMMER FLOW YOGA SEQUENCE *(CONTINUED)*

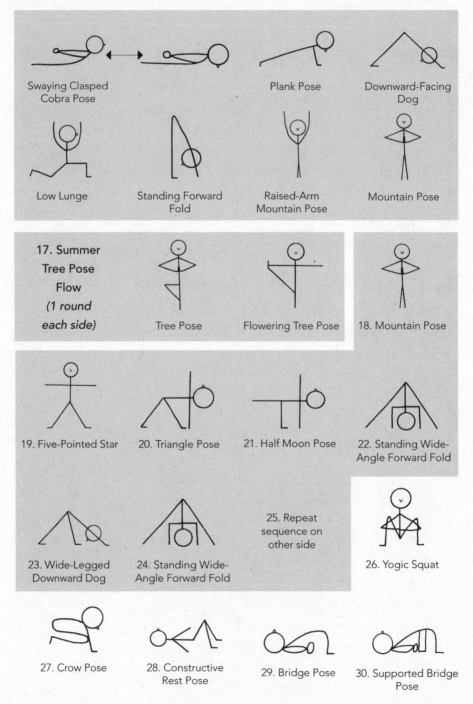

Swaying Clasped
Cobra Pose

Plank Pose

Downward-Facing
Dog

Low Lunge

Standing Forward
Fold

Raised-Arm
Mountain Pose

Mountain Pose

**17. Summer
Tree Pose
Flow
(1 round
each side)**

Tree Pose

Flowering Tree Pose

18. Mountain Pose

19. Five-Pointed Star

20. Triangle Pose

21. Half Moon Pose

22. Standing Wide-
Angle Forward Fold

23. Wide-Legged
Downward Dog

24. Standing Wide-
Angle Forward Fold

25. Repeat
sequence on
other side

26. Yogic Squat

27. Crow Pose

28. Constructive
Rest Pose

29. Bridge Pose

30. Supported Bridge
Pose

SUMMER FLOW YOGA SEQUENCE *(CONTINUED)*

31. Supported Shoulder Stand

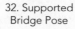

32. Supported Bridge Pose

33. Bridge Pose

34. Constructive Rest Pose

35. Wheel Pose or Bridge Pose

36. Constructive Rest Post

37. Eye of the Needle Pose

38. One-Knee Spinal Twist

39. Happy Baby Pose

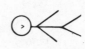

40. Final Relaxation

41. Cooling Breath

42. Compassion Meditation

43. Dedication of Merit

arch into Cow Pose. As you exhale, take your hips back to your heels into Child's Pose. Move back and forth between these two shapes five times.

4. *Lion's Roar* (1 minute): After your fifth time in Child's Pose, inhale back to your hands and knees. Stay there. Now take a big inhalation, and as you exhale, arch your spine, look up between your eyebrows, open your mouth really wide, and stretch your tongue out, as if you were trying to stretch the tip of your tongue to your chin. Let out an "ahhhh" sound from deep in your belly. Really roar! Repeat this three times to release any pent-up tension or aggression.

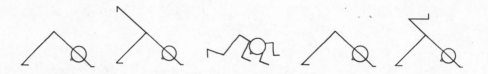

5. *Downward-Facing Dog* (5 to 10 breaths): See page 118.
6. *Three-Legged Dog* (5 breaths): Inhale and lift up your left leg. Keep your hips level.
7. *Deep Lunge* (5 breaths): As you exhale, swing your left leg forward, your foot landing between your hands. Lower your back knee to the ground. Walk your hands to the inside of your front foot, aiming your chest and belly over to the right. Stay up on your palms, or lower down to your forearms. Relax your head. When you've finished, step back to Downward-Facing Dog, and repeat on the other side.
8. *Downward-Facing Dog* (5 breaths).
9. *Three-Legged Dog with Bent Leg* (5 breaths): Repeat the Three-Legged Dog, but this time open up your left hip rather than keeping it square with the right, and bend your knee.

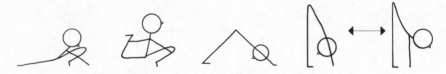

10. *Pigeon Pose* (5 breaths): See page 111.
11. *Pigeon Pose Thigh Stretch* (5 breaths): From Pigeon Pose, inhale and lift your chest up to vertical. Stretch your right arm back behind you, and bend your right leg in toward your buttocks. Take hold of your right foot with your right hand, and swivel your torso forward, becoming square with the hips again. Keep guiding your foot in toward your buttocks as the foot resists back and kicks into your hand. When you've finished, come back to Downward-Facing Dog and repeat on the other side.
12. *Downward-Facing Dog* (5 breaths).
13. *Standing Forward Fold Flow* (5 times): From Downward-Facing Dog, walk your feet forward to your hands until they're outer hip width apart. Inhale, and take your hands to your shins, extend your spine, and look up, coming into ½ Standing Forward Fold. Exhale, and lengthen the crown of your head down toward your feet. Flow up and down.

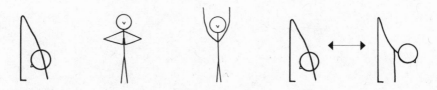

14. *Standing Forward Fold* (5 breaths).

15. *Mountain Pose* (5 breaths): Still folding forward, exhale and take your hands to your hips, and inhaling, come up to stand. Bring your hands in front of your heart to prayer position. Return to your three-part breath, flowing through you like water. Feel your feet, relax your eyes. Inhale the colors, sounds, textures, and smells all around you.

16. *Moon Salutations* (3 times on each side)

    • *Mountain Pose.*

    • *Raised-Arm Mountain Pose:* Inhale, stretch your arms all the way up, and look up and arch back.

    • *Standing Forward Fold Flow* (5 breaths): Exhale and fold forward. Inhale and look up; exhale and fold in.

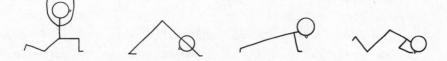

    • *Low Lunge* (5 breaths). Inhale and step your left leg back. Exhale and lower your left knee to the ground. Inhale and sweep your arms out and up and arch back.

    • *Downward-Facing Dog* (5 breaths): Exhale, and step back to Downward-Facing Dog.

    • *Plank Pose* (5 breaths): Inhale and bring your shoulders forward over your wrists.

    • *Modified Push-Up:* Exhale and lower knees, chest, and chin to the ground.

    • *Swaying Clasped Cobra Pose:* Inhale and stretch your legs back behind you and interlace your fingers behind your back. Rise up as you inhale, and lower down as you exhale four times. On your fifth time up, hold for 5 breaths.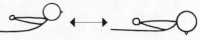

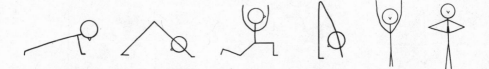

- *Plank Pose:* Inhale back up to Plank Pose.
- *Downward-Facing Dog* (5 breaths): Exhale into Downward-Facing Dog.
- *Low Lunge* (5 breaths): Inhale, and step your left foot forward between your hands. Exhale as you lower the right knee down. Inhale and sweep your arms out to the sides and then overhead and arch back.
- *Standing Forward Fold* (5 breaths): Exhale, lower your hands down, and step your back foot forward.
- *Raised-Arm Mountain Pose:* Inhale and sweep your arms out to the sides and then overhead.
- *Mountain Pose* (5 breaths): Exhale and move your hands in front of your heart in prayer position. Repeat again on the right side. Do one more round (left and right) with this same breath count, and one final round (left and right) with one breath for each posture. Finish in Mountain Pose.

17. *Summer Tree Pose Flow*
- *Tree Pose* (5 to 10 breaths): From Mountain Pose, shift your weight onto your left foot. Lift your right foot up, and bring it to the inside of your left thigh. Bring your hands in front of your heart. *Beginners:* For help with balance, you can hold on to a wall for support, or begin gradually by putting the right toes on the ground and bringing the heel into the left inner ankle. *Advanced students:* Lift your arms overhead and open them out into a wide V, imagining that you're blossoming like your favorite tree. Look up.
- *Flowering Tree Pose:* From Tree Pose, hook your right hand under your right thigh, releasing your right foot away from your left leg. Beginning students can stay here. If you want to go further, take hold of your right big toe with your "peace fingers" (or use a strap as an arm extender and stretch the leg out to the side). Stand upright and stretch your left arm out to the side. Blossom open. For an extra challenge, look up. Return to Mountain Pose. Repeat on the other side.

18. *Mountain Pose* (5 breaths).

19. *Five-Pointed Star* (5 breaths): Step your left foot out to the left so all ten toes are pointing forward. Keep the outer edges of your feet parallel, with about one leg's distance between your feet. Stretch your arms straight out to your sides, palms facing down. Stretch out through the five points of your star: your arms, your legs, and your spine.

20. *Triangle Pose* (5 breaths): See page 122. Begin on the left side. *Advanced students:* Wrap your top arm behind you, and take hold of your front thigh to roll your top shoulder more open as you look up.

21. *Half Moon Pose* (5 breaths): From Triangle Pose, bend your left knee. Touch your left fingertips to the ground (or block) a few inches forward of your left baby toe. Inhale and lift your right leg up, bringing it parallel with your torso. Flex your toes back. *Beginners:* You can place your  right hand on your hip, your left hand on a block, and look down. *Advanced students:* You can stretch your right arm up to the ceiling and look up, bend the back leg, hold the ankle with your top hand, and curl your chest and face open to the sky.

22. *Standing Wide-Angle Forward Fold* (5 breaths): From Half Moon Pose, reach the top leg down and come back through Triangle Pose for a breath. Then bring the outer edges of your feet parallel and fold forward between your legs. Bring the heels of your hands in line with your heels, fingers facing forward. Keep drawing your shoulder blades up toward your hips. *Note:* For beginners and in cases of sciatica, injured hamstrings, and tight hips and backs, keep your knees bent.

23. *Wide-Legged Downward Dog* (5 breaths): Now walk your hands forward, keeping them shoulder width apart, and come into a Wide-Legged Downward Dog.

24. *Standing Wide-Angle Forward Fold* (5 breaths): Walk your hands back to this position again.

25. From Five-Pointed Star, repeat the rest of the sequence on the other side. Finish in Standing Wide-Angle Forward Fold.

26. *Yogic Squat* (5 breaths): Toe-heel your feet in so that your feet are a little wider than hip width apart, and bend your knees down into a squat. You can turn your feet out slightly. If your heels don't come to the ground, place a rolled blanket underneath them. Put your hands in prayer position with your elbows on the insides of your knees. Keep lifting and widening your chest.

27. *Crow Pose* (5 breaths): From Yogic Squat, lean forward and place your palms down flat on the ground, shoulder width apart. Spread your fingers wide apart. Lift up your heels, and place your knees on your triceps. Now lift your feet up as you also lift your chest. Look at the floor a few feet in front of your hands, spread your toes, and bring your feet together and up toward your hips. You can round your back here, like a parachute.

    Tip: Keep a light and playful attitude as you practice. To help with this, smile as you go. Think of a Buddha smile. Exude a quiet contentment, and don't take yourself too seriously!

28. *Constructive Rest Pose* (5 to 10 breaths): From Crow Pose, lie down on your back and let your breath slow down and become even again. See page 125.

29. *Bridge Pose* (5 breaths): See page 125.

30. *Supported Bridge Pose* (1 to 3 minutes): Place a block underneath your sacrum, oriented perpendicular to your spine, at the height that's most comfortable for your lower back, then come into Bridge Pose and rest with the three-part breath. See page 166.

31. *Supported Shoulder Stand* (1 to 3 minutes): From Supported Bridge Pose, lift your feet off the ground, and stretch them up to the ceiling. When you've finished, carefully bend your knees and return one foot down to the ground at a time.

32. *Supported Bridge Pose* (5 to 10 breaths).

33. *Bridge Pose* (5 breaths).

34. *Constructive Rest Post* (5 breaths).

35. *Wheel Pose* or *Bridge Pose* (5 breaths): Place your hands next to your ears. Keep your wrists parallel with the top end of your mat, your fingertips pointing back toward your feet, elbows over wrists. Place your knees over your ankles and your feet hip width apart. Inhale, and press up onto the crown of your head. Draw your elbows over your wrists. Exhale here, and on the inhale, come   up. Make sure that you also keep drawing your knees together so that your thighs remain parallel. Look down at the mat between your hands. Come out slowly, rolling your spine down from top to bottom. *Advanced students:* You can repeat the Wheel Pose up to 3 to 6 times.

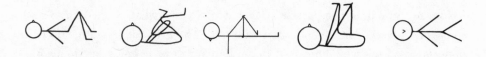

36. *Constructive Rest Pose* (5 breaths).
37. *Eye of the Needle Pose* (5 breaths): Begin with your left leg on top. See page 111.
38. *One-Knee Spinal Twist* (5 breaths): Begin to the left. See page 112.
39. *Happy Baby Pose* (5 breaths): Widen your knees, and lift up your feet until your shins are perpendicular to the ground. Flex your feet, and hold on to the insides of them, drawing your knees down toward your armpits. Keep your sacrum on the ground. Finish by drawing your knees in toward your chest.
40. *Final Relaxation* (5 to 10 minutes): See page 126.
41. *Cooling Breath* (5 minutes): Come to a comfortable seated posture. Rest with your palms facing up on your thighs. Close your eyes. Bring your attention to your nostrils. Feel the breath flowing in and out of them. Now imagine that you're inhaling cool air and a sense of deep contentment and joy, only through your left nostril. Then imagine that you're exhaling warm air and any resentment or agitation through your right nostril and returning it to the earth. Continue like this for a few more minutes, inhaling through the left and exhaling through the right.
42. *Compassion Meditation* (5 to 30 minutes): Read instructions on page 77.
43. *Dedication of Merit* (1 minute): Please review instructions on page 52.

MINI-SUMMER FLOW PRACTICE

If you're short on time, you can do this one in fifteen to twenty minutes:

- Moon Salutations (2 complete rounds)
- Triangle Pose and Half Moon Pose (both sides)
- Standing Wide-Angle Forward Fold
- Supported Bridge and Shoulder Stand
- Eye of the Needle (both sides)
- Happy Baby Pose
- Final Relaxation (2 to 3 minutes)

COMPASSION MEDITATION

Before my grandmother passed away I never knew what it felt like to lose someone I loved so much and was so close to. The grief, depression, and out-of-sorts-ness I felt were immense. I found it hard to work and relate to people. Some of my friends could handle it, but others couldn't. I found that the difference between these two camps was that the former had known deep loss and the latter hadn't. The former could relate to my pain and hold space for me without needing to fix or take care of me. My tears and melancholy didn't make them uncomfortable, for they had sat with that same discomfort. This is compassion.

Compassion is being able to stay open and present to another's suffering — without numbing out or getting so absorbed in her experience that you lose yourself. It takes courage to cultivate compassion, courage to face the pain and suffering both within yourself and in another. The benefits are worth it, though, for compassion is a tremendously powerful force for healing, forgiving, and serving others. It's what allowed the Dalai Lama to forgive the Chinese persecutors who exiled him from his homeland or what calls a mother to, in time, forgive the man who shot her son.

The first step toward feeling authentic, loving warmth for another, even in the face of deep hurt, requires first feeling it for oneself. Cultivating passion for yourself requires patience, courage, and curiosity. When you sit with any emotion long enough — rather than running as fast as you can in the opposite direction — even the hardest one to feel can land you right in the center of your heart. And that's exactly where you find compassion. How do you treat yourself when you know you've made a mistake? Do you beat yourself up for it? Indulge in self-criticism? Or touch your heart and like a loving mother say,

"Sweet girl, it's okay. You messed up. You didn't mean to do that. But it's okay. I forgive you. Let's learn from this and start again."

The more I rest with my own discomfort and pain the more I am able to do that for others without trying to fix them or solve their problems. I can be a loving witness. But it must start in me. An innately feminine quality, compassion allows you to stay grounded in yourself, in your heart, while feeling not only yourself but also another very deeply.

Compassion's final stage is action. We hold space — for ourselves or another — and then act in service of our heart's stirrings. That's what allowed Julia Butterfly Hill to fight for her beloved redwoods, Mahatma Gandhi to lead his homeland to freedom through nonviolence, or you to pick up this book and make some loving changes in your life.

Here's a meditation practice to help you cultivate compassion:

1. Sit in a comfortable position. Close your eyes. Bring your attention to your natural breathing. Relax into its rhythm and how it feels in your body.

2. Now imagine that there's a big, open window in the middle of your chest. You can imagine any kind of window you want — big panes, shutters, you name it. See what's on either side of that window: the vast, limitless space of your heart on one side and the big, open blue sky on the other.

3. As you inhale, let all that you're feeling and experiencing (thoughts, emotions, sensations) enter in through that window. Invite them into your open heart. Hug the such-ness of this moment to you.

4. As you exhale, breathe it all back out through the window into wide-open space with no obstruction or resistance.

5. Continue this way for about five more minutes, or as long as you feel comfortable. Everything is welcome to move in and out. Resist nothing, reject nothing, cling to nothing. Hold your center and your solid ground while inviting life to flow through you. You can end here or continue by adapting this practice to serve someone in your life who needs your compassion. As you inhale, embrace that person's experience in your heart, and as you exhale, send her light, love, and spaciousness.

6. To finish your practice, return to Mindfulness Meditation for a minute or two. Then bring your hands to your heart and dedicate the merit of your practice to the benefit of all beings. Bow toward your heart and, with care and presence, return to your day. *Tip:* A simple way to touch into compassion for yourself throughout your day, whenever you're feeling challenged, is to place one hand on your heart, close your eyes, and take a few deep

breaths, feeling your own loving touch. You can even say to yourself (silently or out loud), "Everything's okay. I love you. I'm here for you."

TRY THIS

Here's another meditation practice that you can try, in addition to your Compassion and Mindfulness Meditations.

Since summer is the shoeless season, try a walking meditation outside in your bare feet. Do it on the grass or the beach. You can even practice it inside (or in the airport when you're waiting for your delayed flight). Stand steady on both feet. Now the object of your meditation is not your breath but what you feel through your feet. As you lift up one foot, say silently to yourself, "lifting." As you move it forward say, "moving," as you place it down on the ground say, "placing," and as you step it down, from the heel to the ball, say, "stepping." Then repeat with the other foot, "lifting," "moving," "placing," "stepping." All you need is a straight line (about twelve to twenty-four feet or so). You can pace forward and back for five to fifteen minutes.

Now let's journey a little bit farther inside yourself to explore how this quality of compassion — as well as the larger gifts of the summer season, such as joy, sensuality, celebration, and connection — has matured in your inner and outer worlds.

REMEMBER

- Practice yoga outdoors this summer to participate in the season's beauty.
- Focus on what feels good in your body as you move and breathe.
- Use your yin practice to cool your system — both in lowering your body temperature and in balancing fiery states such as agitation and overdoing.
- Practice flow yoga in the morning or evening, with a slow tempo and even breath. Have fun with it. Keep it light.
- Cultivate compassion to keep your heart open in the face of your own and others' pain.

Chapter 13

SUMMER REFLECTIONS

By this time, halfway through the year, you've probably noticed how many different moods you've experienced. On some days you've felt like you were breathing fire, wanting to ignite anyone who got in your way. On others you felt like you could do anything, that you were beautiful, and that life was on your side. And you've had days when your heart felt so heavy you thought you'd never taste joy again. And around and around you go. Around and around we all go, through so many different seasons of our hearts and lives.

To help you reflect on what you've learned through your brave participation in all these practices, let's take some time now to notice all that has transpired over the past few months. Since summer is the season to receive and celebrate, find simple ways to honor your accomplishments.

MIDYEAR REFLECTIONS

It's good to revisit our goals and dreams regularly, both to stay inspired and to revamp them as needed to suit our changing lives. Take a look at the intentions that you set for our year together in chapter 5. Then write responses to the following questions:

1. From my list of what I longed to see, be, or, experience this year, _____ has come to fruition, and I (did or will) celebrate this by _____.

2. Of my top three spiritual goals for this year, I have (or would still like to) _____, and I (did or will) celebrate this by _____.

3. Of my top three professional goals for this year, I have (or would still like to) _____, and I (did or will) celebrate this by _____.

4. Of my top three personal/family/community goals for this year, I have (or would still like to) _____, and I (did or will) celebrate this by _____.

5. Of my top three health goals for this year, I have (or would still like to) _____, and I (did or will) celebrate this by _____.

6. Out of all of my aspirations for this year, I'm realizing that I need to let go of _____ because _____.

7. Out of all of my aspirations for this year, I'm most interested in realizing _____, _____, and _____. I could use the support of _____ and _____ to help me do that.

SUMMER REFLECTIONS

Now, looking back over the past season, take an honest look at how things have been for you, in both your outer and inner experiences, and explore them in your journal through the questions below.

MONTH ONE

1. At the start of this season, I felt most agitated and stressed by:
2. My main health concerns were:
3. The three main ways that I sabotaged my own pleasure, playfulness, and enjoyment were:
4. The part of myself or my life that was the most challenging to celebrate was:
5. The one habit I'm going to really focus on cultivating for the next thirty days is _____. I will omit _____ in order to create space for this. The main things I hope to experience as a result of this are:

MONTH TWO

1. My inner life has become more colorful this season through _____ and _____. My outer life has become more colorful this season through _____ and _____. The results I'm feeling are mostly _____ and _____.
2. The three words I'd use to describe my connection with my sexuality right now are _____, _____, and _____. Ideally, those three words would be _____, _____, and _____.

3. I'm showing compassion for myself by _____, and I'm showing it for others by _____.
4. What's brought me the most joy this month is:
5. When I feel angry and agitated, my default reaction is to _____. Some other more skillful responses that I want to explore are _____ and _____.

MONTH THREE

1. What I'm celebrating most from my efforts this season are:
2. Looking back, I realize that my biggest challenges were:
3. I'm feeling called to put my compassion into action by donating my money or time and services to:
4. When I think back to the times when I was the most playful, the following memories come to mind:
5. Some ways that I'm practicing receiving include:

COMMUNITY RITUAL

Invite your partner or children to come to the farmers' market with you. Make a morning of it, then stay and have lunch there. Take your children or nieces and nephews to a paint-your-own-pottery studio. You can also gather your girlfriends for a summer solstice ritual or to spend a weekend at the beach or a day at the pool. Get out and enjoy the colors of life together.

The more fully we experience life's beauty, the less regret we have that we didn't live and love in the way that we most longed to. As the summer sun starts to wane and ease into the golden light of autumn, we're faced with the inevitable impermanence of life. Leaves begin to decay down to their skeletons, and it's time for us too to let go with grace. Let's step into the autumn now and see what wisdom she has to reveal to us.

PART 4

AUTUMN

Element: METAL

Color: WHITE

Organs: LUNGS AND LARGE INTESTINE

Heart qualities: SORROW, COURAGE, AND JOY

Life cycle: MID- TO LATE ADULTHOOD

Creative cycle: HARVESTING AND FEASTING

Menstrual cycle: THE WEEK BEFORE MENSTRUATION

Moon cycle: WANING MOON

Actions: GATHERING, FOCUSING, TURNING INWARD,
AND LETTING GO

Focus: RECEIVE THE GROWTH YOU'VE EXPERIENCED
FROM THE PAST SIX MONTHS, AND LET GO OF WHAT NO LONGER
SERVES YOU. TAKE WITH YOU ONLY WHAT YOU NEED.

Chapter 14

HARVESTING

Autumn is my favorite time of the year, perhaps because I grew up in Connecticut surrounded by the splendor of changing leaves. The season's crisp winds, golden light, and first days of school instill a fresh, buzzing, alive feeling inside. I feel inspired to complete unfinished projects before the holidays, and I love bringing out cuddly winter sweaters, woolly scarves, and cozy tights. Long walks through crinkly leaves remind me of romping in leaf piles on my way home from school as a young girl.

The magic of the season extends deeper than our wardrobes, though, for during these crucial months, nature prepares for her long winter's rest and teaches us to do the same. It is time to gather, store, organize, and wind down from summer's high tempo and the relentless forward momentum that modern living usually demands. When the crisp winds of autumn start to blow, we need to tune in to the signal that it's time to start slowing down. As leaves fall to the ground, they decay and merge with the earth once again. We too are in the process of letting things wither and fall away to gather only what is essential for the winter months. We're reminded that, eventually, we have to let go of *everything* in order to die countless little deaths in each of our lifetimes, and this ultimately prepares us for the final letting.

Beginning with the fall equinox on September 21 (March 21 in the southern hemisphere), when the dark and the light live in equal measure, the days grow shorter and shorter until the longest night of the year arrives with the winter solstice. In the Jewish tradition Rosh Hashanah calls in the new year, and for Muslims Ramadan is the holiest point in the year, a time to purify and strengthen connection to God. Hindus mark the coming of winter with Narvatri, or "the nine nights of the goddess."

Just as people of these faiths step out of their lives to pray and honor the larger cycles of life, we too intuitively respond to this season's changes by spending more time at home with our families and immersed in projects and study. This contracting quality draws us not only into our homes but also deeper into our inner, emotional worlds — a big difference from the playful, carefree exuberance of summer. Now's the time to reap the benefits from the past six months and appreciate all the ways you've grown and flowered. It's time to start spending more time alone to see how those outward expansions translate to your inner spiritual and creative life. What's essential? What will you take with you into the dreamtime of the winter, and what will you leave behind?

THE METAL ELEMENT

Metal, the dominant element of this season, comes forth from the ashen earth of late summer and into form through the alchemy of reduction and refinement until it glistens pure and unpolluted. This season we become the alchemists of our own change. Like metal, we evolve through reduction. What needs to be removed and stripped away so that the glistening essence of who we are can shine like a diamond?

> ### TRY THIS
>
> List five projects that you've put on the back burner and want to focus on for the next few months. Then, underneath these, write down the action steps that you need to take to make them happen.

This paring down comes through discernment and faith. Take an honest look at yourself and your life. What's working? What's not? What can you let go of on your own, and with what do you need guidance? Traditional Chinese Medicine acknowledges that grief and sadness are the primary emotions of the autumn season, which, when tended to, are transmuted into courage. The lung and the large intestine are the activated organs that work together, receiving and releasing — oxygen and carbon dioxide in the lungs, and water, nutrients, and waste in the large intestine. Both provide crucial life-giving energy through this powerful interchange. They too are alchemists, taking in what is needed to shine and letting go of whatever might hold us back. When this pair is weakened through stress, unexpressed emotions, poor breathing, pollution, smoking, or toxic diets, things get stuck. And feelings of immobilization, depression, and suppressed grief can intensify and rock you off center.

LETTING GO

Letting go is perhaps one of life's most difficult lessons to learn. However, it's the most crucial one, for everything in our lives, big and small, withers away to one degree or another. At some point we're all going to have to say good-bye to everything and everyone that we love. The question is, then, how gracefully can you let go? How much can you give in to the way things are? How well can you honor yourself and that which is passing?

Considering the immense anxiety, fear, and sadness that we experience with even the *thought* of letting go of something we love, we can start to learn this lesson in simple, more manageable situations, such as our own breathing. With each cycle of breath, you're letting go. Every time you fall asleep at night, your body surrenders deeply. When you're entrenched in an argument with your daughter and choose to relinquish your stubborn position, you're letting go.

In your colon, constipation can be a sign that you're too tightly wound, trying to control your surroundings so that you don't have to surrender. Making larger changes in your life — that reveal your trust for the way things are — can help your body find its natural state of ease and flow. Sometimes you need to let things wither away, like summer's blossoms, before you can start on something new. Can you let yourself rest with reality, even if it's not how you want it to be? Can you trust the larger timing and wisdom behind everything?

> ## TRY THIS
>
> Write a letter to something or someone you're ready to let go of. As you write, keep in mind that there's no need to mail it. In fact, I encourage you not to, so you can feel free to write what's most true for you. Instead, when you've finished, make a ritual of burning it on the new moon.
>
> Write all the things you've learned from this person or experience. Although some of these lessons may have been unsavory, record how they have helped you to become the person you are right now. If it feels right, write down any blessings or well wishes as you release him/her/it. Tell him or her what you are carrying with you as you move forward and that it's time for you to leave him or her behind.

Letting go also means allowing yourself to be completely as you are and to do whatever you need to do to loosen your grip. Sometimes, to do this, you need to let yourself feel completely out of control. We see this when we witness a friend experiencing tremendous grief. We hold space for her to wail, sleep all day, rant and rave, or do whatever she needs to do to move the energy of her pain and, in turn, move on. The process isn't always pretty, but it's real. Letting go asks us to be ruthlessly candid about what we feel and how much we have loved.

Take a good look at what relationships, beliefs, and activities no longer serve you. You will see where you are ready to let go, and you can use the currents of saying good-bye and grieving inherent in this season to lead you gracefully to where new opportunities, people, and ways of being await.

Leaning into unsavory feelings doesn't mean that you're a miserable, pessimistic person who sabotages her happiness — just the opposite. Diving into the discomfort brings you directly into your heart and into a deep, abiding joy that's always your essence and doesn't depend on your mood or on whether or not things are going your way. This is what the alchemy of the season teaches us: to strip away what is nonessential to reveal what is true and everlasting.

While the long-term repercussions of repressing emotion can manifest as disease, the short-term signs that you're not honoring your feelings are anxiety and too much mental stimulation. This can make you feel a lot like the Energizer Bunny — always staying in motion to avoid any kind of intimacy with yourself. This constant motion, along with a failure to rest and nurture yourself, keeps you from tasting the bliss that comes when you face yourself completely.

STAYING GROUNDED

When I met Colleen several years ago, she was a student at my teacher training in Thailand. Colleen had struggled with staying grounded amid all the changes she was going through during this intensive month-long course. Colleen was thin, agile, and hypersensitive, and her mind and body harbored a predominance of the air element in Ayurveda, which is more prone to disturbance in the autumn. When in balance, she exuded creativity and spiritual devotion; when out of balance, anxiety, confusion, and insomnia (all pointing to overactivity in the "air" of the mind) plagued her.

These latter imbalances resurfaced in Thailand, to the point where Colleen had hardly slept for the entire thirty-day course. Try rubbing sesame oil on your feet and head before bed, I had coaxed. Drink hot milk with nutmeg before bed. I had offered her remedy after remedy, yet nothing seemed to work. She couldn't find a way to befriend her anxiety, to just rest with it. And the more it persisted, the more she resisted it. And the more wound up she became.

Then, about three weeks into the training, something shifted. Her tissues began to look softer, shedding their steely vigilance. Her skin took on more of a dewy glow. She sat relaxed, yet joyfully engaged. The previous few nights, she said, she was able to bring to bed the loving, aware presence that we had spoken of and worked with so often.

"It was like I was with my little girl," she explained, "only I was the mother *and* the little girl. I was able to accept my discomfort, my fatigue, my anxiety, and to feel love and compassion for myself, as I usually do for my daughter. Then, before I knew it, I was asleep. That night taught me how to be with myself — off the mat and off the cushion."

Before Colleen returned home to New England, she asked for some advice about readjusting to the cold, autumn temperatures there while maintaining the positive shifts she had experienced in Thailand. Together we looked at her diet and daily schedule to see what needed to shift in order for her to get grounded in her home climate as the air got dryer and the temperatures started to plummet. When she arrived home she started to wake up with the sun, then spent ten minutes in a breath-centered, seated meditation. Then she enjoyed a slow, mindful yoga practice or walk through the forest. These simple shifts helped her to harmonize her scattered and erratic inner world with the steadiness of her environment. She used the practices I've outlined about relaxing before bedtime too. In this way, Colleen could keep her center while participating in her ups and downs, as she had learned to do on those last nights in Thailand.

AUTUMN RITUALS

As the days grow shorter, it's perfectly okay to allow yourself more time to rest since your circadian rhythm is shifting, along with the earth's. This could mean going to sleep a little earlier, waking up a little later, even taking a catnap in the afternoon. You'll also want to replace the coconut oil you used for self-massage during the summertime with sesame oil (heated up), which is more warming and insulating.

During the day, ask yourself, "How can I work smarter, not harder? Where can I ask for help from others? What can I delegate? What's simply wasting my time?" Let yourself know that it's perfectly okay to take little pleasure breaks in the midst of tasks. If you've blocked off two hours to finish writing that report that's due tomorrow, every twenty-five minutes stand up, place your feet hip width apart, put your hands on your hips, and circle them wide, drawing figure eights with them. Step outside for some fresh air. Turn on some Michael Jackson, and have a mini–dance party with yourself. Find ways to bring doses of fun into this more contracted, introverted, and productive season.

A friend of mine involves her daughter in celebrating autumn by leaving an offering plate full of treats — a pear, chestnuts, pumpkin, or pomegranate — outside under a tree for the "autumn fairies." The next morning they hunt in the yard for the gift of the fairies: a basket of fall goodies. There are countless more ways to celebrate this season. Indulge in quiet walks, but when you go out be sure to keep your head and neck warm since your immunity is quite compromised this time of the year. Sip warm drinks. Take hot baths with lavender oil. Now's the time to safeguard your health to keep your immunity strong through the approaching cold and hectic holiday season. Let yourself cry when you need to. Turn to the healing power of prayer and ask for guidance, support, and protection during painful transitions. Let it be okay if you're less social than usual. Spend more time getting to know yourself again. Infuse your home or bath (or adorn your body) with essential oils of sandalwood, vetiver, neroli, and geranium. Light candles or a fire inside — or even better, sit at a bonfire outside with friends — and release whatever you need to let go of into the flames.

THE DAILY SELF-MASSAGE WITH OIL

This ancient, Ayurvedic practice is beneficial any day of the year — but it's even more so in the autumn because of its capacity to ground, warm, and calm during an otherwise cold and dry season. It's also helpful for cleansing (done regularly during Ayurvedic detoxification programs called Panchakarma) because it draws toxins out of the tissues and into the bloodstream for elimination. Ideally, the whole process takes about ten minutes. You can indulge in this once a week or during the one-day seasonal retreat. Otherwise, every day, you can just oil up and then get in the shower. Here's how to do it:

1. Warm up about a quarter cup of organic sesame oil. Be sure it's not too hot. It should be comfortable enough to go directly on your skin.
2. Massage the oil into your body, starting with your head (including in your hair if you'll be washing it), around your ears and face. Then work downward to your feet, paying extra attention to your belly (use a circular motion there) and the soles of your feet. Use long, smooth strokes on your limbs and circles on your joints.
3. Sit on the edge of your tub, or sit or lie down on a towel on the floor. Relax and breathe deeply for ten minutes while the oil sinks in. Then take a hot shower or bath, washing the oil off with a gentle soap.

THE ONE-DAY AUTUMN LETTING-GO RETREAT

If you find it challenging to incorporate all of this season's rituals regularly, try this one-day retreat. Autumn, like the spring, is a potent time for cleansing. This one-day sojourn will help you to shed all that you don't need, both physically and emotionally. To prepare, remember to find a quiet space. Go to a hotel or a B and B for a day, or stay at a friend's house if she has gone out of town. Also, make yourself a pot of *kitchari* (recipe on page 203) before you start. Remember to completely unplug today: turn off your phone and computer, and practice a day of silence.

- Let yourself sleep in for as long as you need to. You'll most likely feel more tired than usual this season, so let yourself catch up on rest.
- Before you get up, remember the preciousness of your life. How lucky are you to be alive? How would you live this day if it were your last?
- Scrape your tongue, brush your teeth, and use your neti pot.
- Drink one or two glasses of warm water with lemon, followed by a cup of ginger tea (recipe on page 260).
- Sit for ten or more minutes in Mindfulness Meditation (page 44).
- Do the autumn yin yoga sequence (page 211).
- Have another glass of warm or hot water with lemon.
- Brush your skin (page 83), and give yourself a massage with sesame oil (page 190). Take a hot shower or bath, followed by a short cold blast.
- Eat a bowl of *kitchari* for breakfast. You can add some ghee (clarified butter) to this if you'd like.
- Enjoy a cup of ginger tea.
- Choose a comfortable place, and write in your journal for thirty minutes. Use some of the journaling topics from page 230, or write three or more pages about whatever feels true for you today.
- Go for a long walk — about an hour. Before you start, look up to the sky and thank it for its inspiration. Look down to the earth,

and thank it for its support. Ask them to help you on your journey of letting go. During the first half of the walk, with each step recall the things you're ready to let go of. During the second half of the walk, with each step, name the things you're ready to take with you into the darkest days of the year. When you've finished, again thank the earth and the sky for their help in your evolution.

- Drink a tall glass of warm or hot water with lemon.
- Sit for ten minutes in Mindfulness Meditation.
- Prepare a bowl of *kitchari* for lunch, adding some steamed vegetable with lemon, if you'd like, followed by a cup of ginger tea.
- Lie down and rest or nap for thirty minutes.
- Choose a spiritually oriented book (see suggestions on my website) to read for the next hour. Drink another glass of warm water.
- Since autumn is also the season to honor our ancestors (read more about this on page 229), now is a good time to gather pictures or mementos from your ancestors. Reflect on the qualities they embodied that you would like to call into your life. Make a place for these photographs or keepsakes on your altar, and light a candle in your ancestors' honor. Pray to them for support and guidance.
- Sit for ten minutes in the Joy Meditation (page 226).
- Do the fall flow yoga practice (page 214).
- Prepare another bowl of *kitchari* for dinner.
- Write the letting-go letter described earlier in this chapter. Light a candle or a fire in your fireplace. Read the letter aloud, and then release it into the flames.
- Take a hot bath with eucalyptus essential oil, with candles lit and some relaxing music playing. Focus on taking deep breaths and feeling supported by the soft strength of the water.
- Sit for ten minutes in Mindfulness Meditation.
- In your journal, name all the things you're grateful for today.
- Make yourself a cup of hot rice or almond milk with a little bit of nutmeg.
- Read your book for a little while, if you like.
- 10:00 P.M.: Lights out!

TRY THIS

When I use the word *prayer*, I'm referring to an open, direct line of communication between your heart and the larger universal heart — whether that's the Divine Mother, God, or any other magnificent force that humbles and inspires you. Prayer's an essential part of any woman's life. It drops her directly into her devotional nature and out of her head. It's here to remind you that you're not in control. That it's okay to surrender. That it's okay to ask for and receive support.

1. Pray anytime, anywhere. I especially invoke the power of prayer when I'm in the midst of a challenge, but you can also use it in very ordinary moments, such as when you're looking for a parking space or wanting to get off the standby list at the airport.
2. Light a candle, or speak to the pictures or figures on your altar. This can help anchor you into the dialogue with either your ancestors or the divine, or both.
3. Speak from your heart. Ask for anything you need help or guidance with. Don't worry about doing it wrong — you can't. Be yourself. Make jokes, if that's your nature. Cry if you're feeling sad. Show up as you are, and know that there's nothing you can't share or ask for.
4. When you're finished say thank you. Ask for signs and synchronicities to show you the way. Affirm that you trust all is working out for your highest good, that you are letting go and leaving the outcome in the hands of the Divine.

AUTUMN MOON TIME PRACTICES

An ancient way to honor your moon time, or the new moon if you're no longer menstruating, is to sleep alone. That's what moon lodges and red tents were for — to help a woman be away from her spouse, her children, and from non-menstruating women to rest in her energy without being drawn outside herself.

Sleeping apart from your partner usually signifies that there's been an argument or a big rift, yet spending time apart can actually be a healthy ritual that supports your relationship. Explain to your partner the larger meaning of your moon time as an opportunity to cleanse, purify, and connect deeply with your spiritual power. Explain that enjoying your own sleeping space will rejuvenate your energy. Spend more time journaling, meditating, and reading inspirational books and poetry before going to bed. Use the solitary space to shed your tears and welcome the changes that are ready to emerge from inside you.

All these practices — slowing down, stripping things away so that you carry with you only what you need, spending more time alone in contemplation, and adjusting your daily rhythm so that you sleep more, are kept warm, and stay close to the earth — help you to weather the demanding life lessons that can blow in with the autumn winds.

REMEMBER

- Spend more time focusing on home and work projects.
- Harvest all your good habits from the past six months. What has served you? Keep those up.
- Allow yourself to cry and grieve when you need to.
- Strengthen your connection to your spirit. Pray, go for quiet walks, give yourself more opportunities to rest.
- Let go of relationships, thoughts, situations, and beliefs that are holding you back.

Chapter 15

IN *the* KITCHEN
Root Wisdom

The other morning I sat at my kitchen table eating breakfast. Looking out the window I watched the first of the season's leaves tumble to the still-green grass. Squirrels scurried around, busily gathering their supplies for winter. Although the convenience of modern living might cause us to temporarily forget, each autumn we too gather nature's bounty in preparation for a long winter's rest.

While we live in an instant-access world where you can go down to your corner grocer and get a peach at the height of winter, now's the time to start eating fewer raw foods and more building foods such as grains, nuts, root vegetables, and seeds. This season's vegetables — such as squashes, pumpkins, beets, and sweet potatoes — grow close to or in the earth, as do nuts and fruits with hard shells, giving us the grounding and stability that our bodies need as the cold winds and the hectic buzz of the holidays arrive.

COMPOSTING

When I lived in Thailand I started a compost pile in my backyard where I could throw all my food scraps. In Boulder the city collects compost along with garbage and recycling, and I keep a small compost bin on my kitchen counter. When you compost your food (not animal meat, though), you're giving it back to the earth to become the nutritive soil from which new food can grow. Consider this: a new study in the American Chemical Society's journal found that Americans waste — just straight-up throw away — the equivalent of 350 million barrels of oil a year in the form of food (that's about seventy times the amount of oil in the BP Gulf oil spill). Let's all start composting![1]

FALL CLEANSING

After spring, fall's the second-best time of year for internal cleansing (see the one-day fall retreat on page 191). Even better, we can do a cleanse in the spring *and* the fall. According to Ayurveda, our health is most vulnerable at the junctions between seasons — those from summer to fall and fall to winter being most sensitive. If there's one season of the year when you should take exceptional care of yourself, this is it. Eating well, resting well, getting appropriate exercise, and sticking to a routine will form the bedrock of your immunity for winter.

I recommend doing an Ayurvedic *kitchari* cleanse in autumn (page 203). Whereas a spring cleanse targets rejuvenating the liver and gallbladder, a fall cleanse treats the lungs and large intestine. The large intestine is perhaps the most taxed organ, owing to the strain we put it under with overeating, especially if we're consuming chemically processed foods. If you're not sure whether your colon's functioning well, here are some clear signs that it is: you're having one to three unstrained bowel movements each day (comes out easily, noiselessly,

---

REMEMBER YOUR RHYTHM

Whereas it feels good to get lackadaisical with our routines and rhythms during the summer, we really need them to find stability in the fall. Establish a regular sleeping, eating, working, resting, and exercise routine. Your body's trying to acclimate to a lot of changes right now, including the weather and new projects, so support her in feeling safe and cared for through establishing healthy rhythms again. Here are topics you can journal about to help you become better acquainted with the rhythms that serve you:

1. Overall, I feel best when I wake up at _____ and go to sleep at _____.
2. The three main things that disrupt this rhythm are:
3. I like to eat breakfast, lunch, and dinner at the following times to feel my best:
4. What gives me the most energy is to exercise on the following days and times:
5. My most creative and productive time of the day is:
6. My least productive and energetic time of the day is _____, and the things to do that don't require a lot of mental energy are _____ and _____.
7. I feel the best when I turn off my computer at _____ and my phone off at _____.
8. The day of the week that I'd most like to regularly rest and unplug is _____.

and in one piece that floats); they're light brown, don't smell much, and are smooth (the consistency of peanut butter); and you're free of gas and bloating.

Signs of colon toxicity include irregular bowel movements, bad breath or body/foot odor, stomach pains, or feeling like you're eating healthy foods but still not being nourished (a sign of poor absorption). If any of these symptoms sound familiar, a colon cleanse will help. In the fall, that includes drinking lots of hot water with lemon (and I also like Yogi DeTox tea), eating high-fiber foods such as whole grains and vegetables, taking colon-cleansing herbs (most contain psyllium husk, and many great formulas can be found in your health food store), and getting colonics or enemas.

NOURISHING AROMAS

Along with routines, the nourishing aromas from a vibrant kitchen also help us to feel safe. These rich, fragrant scents soothe the soul and awaken a primal sense of security and safety.

Smell, the sense most closely related to one of this season's dominant organs, the lungs, is one of the first ways that a food communicates its essence and stimulates our appetite. Also, one of the best ways that you can tell whether a food is spoiled is to smell it. To invite a sense of warmth into your home this season, step into the familiar healing zone that women have owned for millennia — in front of the primal cook fire that is now your stove or oven. Enjoy the goodness your cooking creates in your kitchen and in your home.

AUTUMN SHOPPING LIST

In many places, farmers' markets are at their prime now, packed with the bounty from the spring and summer. It's a great time to bring more of nature inside by storing grains, legumes, dried herbs, and spices in glass jars and arranging them on open shelves in your kitchen, where you can enjoy their colors and textures (and spend less time fishing through crowded cupboards for them). Think of it as your cold-season garden.

The dominant color this season is white (the white from the natural world, not from white flour and sugar), for these white foods best moisturize and strengthen your lungs and large intestine during this dry and often blustery stretch. Some examples of white foods include daikon (a Chinese radish — grate some and put it over your food or add it to soup or *kitchari*), quinoa, millet, amaranth, apples, garlic, ginger, oats, pears, parsnips, turnips, and onions.

Here is a list of all the foods, including the white ones, that will best support you this season:

adzuki beans	kidney beans
amaranth	melons
apples	millet
bananas	mung beans
barley	oats
broccoli	okra
brown rice pasta	onions
Brussels sprouts	parsnips
cabbage	pears
carrots	peppers
cauliflower	persimmons
collard greens	pumpkin
corn	quinoa
cranberries	raisins
daikon	short-grain brown rice
dates	sweet potatoes
eggplant	turnips
figs	wild mushrooms
garlic	wild rice
ginger	yams
greens	

BREAKFAST MENU

- Green Goddess Smoothie
- Apple Walnut Quinoa Porridge

GREEN GODDESS SMOOTHIE

Serves 2

Pear combined with almond milk creates a nice, creamy consistency, while the warming spices of cinnamon and ginger help to rev up circulation and bolster your immune system. And turmeric is a wonderful lung tonic.

3 dates
1 pear, cut and seeded
½ inch peeled fresh ginger, chopped
1 cup almond milk (recipe on page 150)
3 to 5 kale leaves
1 tablespoon brown rice protein powder
1 teaspoon turmeric
dash of cinnamon
spring water, as needed
optional: other superfoods (page 95)

Soak dates in water for 20 minutes, then drain and remove pits. Put dates, pear, ginger, and almond milk in a blender, and blend until smooth. Add the kale, protein powder, turmeric, and cinnamon. Blend until smooth. For a thinner smoothie, add water.

APPLE WALNUT QUINOA PORRIDGE

Serves 2

A warm bowl of porridge feels so soothing and nourishing on cool mornings. Walnuts and flaxseeds, high in omega-3 fatty acids, are also warming and very nutritive for the lungs and large intestine.

1 apple
2 tablespoons freshly ground flaxseeds
1 cup water, rice milk, or almond milk (recipe on page 150)
½ cup quinoa
1 small handful raisins
pinch of cinnamon
pinch of sea salt
1 handful walnuts
raw honey or maple syrup to taste

Shred the apple and place it in a medium bowl with the flaxseeds; set aside. In a saucepan, combine water or milk, quinoa, raisins, cinnamon, and salt, and bring to a boil. Reduce heat and simmer for 15 to 20 minutes, until all the liquid is absorbed. Fluff the quinoa mixture with a fork, add it to the bowl with the apples, and mix. Top with walnuts and honey or syrup.

MORE BREAKFAST IDEAS

- Baked cinnamon raisin or cashew date mochi (pounded sweet brown rice; I like the brand Grainassance) with a little ghee or almond butter.
- Miso soup (recipe on page 256) and brown rice.
- Baked pears with granola (recipe on page 149) and warm almond milk.

LUNCH MENU

- Butternut Squash Curry with Collards and Brown Rice

BUTTERNUT SQUASH CURRY WITH COLLARDS AND BROWN RICE

Serves 4

My years in Asia taught me to love curries in all forms. They're great for the cold-weather months because they heat you up and boost metabolism. Squash is also warming, grounding, and helpful in improving energy circulation.

1 cup brown basmati rice
1-inch piece kombu seaweed*
5 cups water, divided, plus extra for sautéeing
2 medium butternut squashes peeled, halved, and seeded
1 bunch collards
1 large onion cut into large chunks
4 garlic cloves, finely chopped
1 2-inch piece fresh ginger, peeled and finely chopped

---

* You can find kombu in the Asian section of your health food store. It comes in long, hard strips that need a lot of cooking to soften. I always add a strip to grains to help make them more alkaline and therefore more digestible. Plus, cooked kombu is really delicious and is loaded with iron and other wonderful minerals.

2 teaspoons sea salt

1½ tablespoons no-salt-added curry powder

1 tablespoon olive oil or ghee

1 15-oz. can of low-fat organic coconut milk

½ cup fresh cilantro, chopped

Rinse the rice. Add the rice, kombu, and 2 cups water to a pot. Bring to a boil, then reduce heat and simmer for 30 to 45 minutes, until rice is tender. As the rice is cooking, cut the squash into ½-inch pieces. Cut the collards into 2-inch strips. Heat olive oil and sauté onion, garlic, ginger, salt, and curry powder, adding water as needed. Cook, stirring often, until caramelized, or about 6 to 8 minutes. In a large pot, add the sautéed ingredients to the coconut milk and 3 cups water. Add squash, and cover partially. Bring to a boil, reduce heat, and simmer gently 7 or 8 minutes. Stir in the collards, and simmer another 5 to 7 minutes until collards turn bright green and squash and collards are tender. Remove from heat, stir in cilantro, and serve over brown rice.

OPTION: For additional protein, add cubes of tofu, tempeh, chicken, or fish when you add the squash.

MORE LUNCH IDEAS

- For a creamy soup, blend the squash curry (before you add the collards). Serve it with steamed greens or Kale Salad with Sprouts (see recipe page 97).
- Sweet potato fries (cut a sweet potato into match sticks, toss with olive oil and tamari, and bake at 400°F for about 30 minutes) with hummus and steamed broccoli in a bowl.
- Fried rice (use the leftover basmati rice) with tofu, egg, or cashew nuts, some curry powder, olive oil, and whatever veggies you have on hand.

SNACK MENU

- Halloween Snack Mix
- Spiced Apple Cider

HALLOWEEN SNACK MIX

Serves 6

Carving pumpkins for Halloween is a favorite autumn pastime in my family. We always conclude by roasting the seeds and snacking on them for days to come. Pumpkin seeds are higher in protein than other seeds and are loaded with omega-3 fatty acids, zinc, calcium, and B vitamins. Kids love to help out with this snack too.

½ cup raw pumpkin seeds
¼ teaspoon coconut oil, melted
¼ cup raw almonds
¼ cup dried cranberries (unsweetened)
¼ cup cacao nibs, dark chocolate chips, or carob chips
¼ teaspoon cayenne pepper
¼ teaspoon sea salt

In a small bowl, toss pumpkin seeds with coconut oil until coated. Spread seeds in a skillet, and heat over medium-high heat. Shaking the skillet constantly, cook 3 minutes, or until most of the pumpkin seeds swell and pop. Transfer to a bowl. Add the almonds to the skillet. Shaking the skillet constantly, cook 30 seconds, or until golden flecks appear. Transfer to the bowl with the pumpkin seeds. Stir in remaining ingredients and mix thoroughly.

SPICED APPLE CIDER

Serves about 8

Here's an autumn favorite, great for parties or for warming up after a long walk. Plus, you can't beat the enticing aroma of cider cooking on the stove.

½ teaspoon whole allspice
1 teaspoon whole cloves
1 cinnamon stick
2 quarts apple cider
1 large orange, cut into thin slices

Place spices and cider in a large pot. Bring to a boil. Reduce heat and simmer for 15 to 30 minutes. Serve in a mug with an orange slice.

HOLIDAY TREAT

MULLED WINE

Serves 8

For Thanksgiving, instead of Spiced Apple Cider, make this mulled wine to celebrate. It's so festive and so delicious!

1 navel orange
4 cups apple juice or cider
2 tablespoons honey or agave nectar
1 2-inch piece fresh ginger, thinly sliced
6 whole allspice berries
10 cinnamon sticks
1 bottle red wine

With a veggie peeler, zest orange into long strips. In a saucepan, gently simmer the zest, apple juice, honey or agave, ginger, allspice, and 2 cinnamon sticks for 20 minutes. Stir in wine and cook until heated through. Strain. Serve hot, in glass mugs if you have them, with remaining cinnamon sticks.

DINNER MENU

- Mung Bean Kitchari
- Roasted Brussels Sprouts

MUNG BEAN KITCHARI

Serves 8

Kitchari *means "food of the gods" in Sanskrit. Prized as a nourishing and cleansing complete meal in Ayurveda, it has long been a staple in my diet when I'm sick, cleansing, or needing to give my system a break. In India it's served in hospitals and to children and the elderly as easy-to-digest nourishment. Mung beans are high in natural vegetable protein and rich in important minerals. Therefore, this recipe is very good for anyone who is recovering from an illness, fatigued, or having digestive problems. It is also good for general detox at the change of season. You can make a big pot and have it for every meal over two to seven days, along with some steamed vegetables.*

1 cup mung beans, whole or split
12 cups water, divided
6 to 7 cups assorted vegetables (carrots, celery, zucchini, broccoli, etc.)
2 tablespoons ghee
2 onions, chopped
1 2-inch piece ginger root, minced
3 to 4 cloves garlic, minced
1 heaping teaspoon turmeric
1 heaping teaspoon cumin powder
½ teaspoon coriander powder
½ teaspoon black pepper
1 tablespoon sea salt
1 cup brown basmati rice
1-inch piece kombu

Wash mung beans and rinse at least 3 times. If you're using whole beans, soak them overnight in 3 cups water; no need to soak split beans. Clean and coarsely chop vegetables. Heat the ghee in a large frying pan. Add onions, ginger, garlic, spices, pepper, and salt. Sauté over medium-high heat until brown. Put beans, 9 cups water, rice, and kombu in a large pot. Add the ingredients from the skillet and bring to a boil. Lower heat, and cook for another 45 to 60 minutes.

OPTION: Garnish with fresh cilantro.

ROASTED BRUSSELS SPROUTS

Serves 6

An easy side dish to put in the oven while the kitchari'*s cooking on the stove, Brussels sprouts are the kind of veggie you either love or love to hate! I happen to love them. Part of the cabbage family, they contain phytonutrients, which ward off carcinogens and other immune invaders. Brussels sprouts are also an exceptional source of calcium, magnesium, vitamins A and C, and beta-carotene.*

1½ pounds Brussels sprouts
3 tablespoons olive oil
1 teaspoon sea salt
½ teaspoon freshly ground black pepper
2 tablespoons tamari or Bragg's Amino Acids
optional: ½ lemon for juicing

Preheat oven to 400°F. Wash and trim the Brussels sprouts, cutting an X in the base of each one to help the heat enter the center and cook the sprouts evenly. Place trimmed Brussels sprouts in a large bowl. Add the olive oil, salt, pepper, and tamari, and toss it all together with your hands until well coated. Pour onto a baking sheet, and place on center oven rack. Roast for 30 to 45 minutes, shaking pan every 5 to 7 minutes for even browning. Reduce heat if necessary to prevent burning. Brussels sprouts should be dark when done. Squeeze some fresh lemon juice over them if you'd like, and serve immediately.

MORE DINNER IDEAS

- Steam a big pot of vegetables and put them in a blender with broth to make a hot, nourishing soup.
- Have breakfast for dinner with one of this season's breakfast options. I love having mochi or quinoa porridge for dinner!
- Cut a spaghetti squash in half, bake it, and fork out the "spaghetti" and serve with marinara sauce and roasted cubes of tempeh.

DESSERT MENU

- Maple Pumpkin Pie

MAPLE PUMPKIN PIE

Serves 8

Thanks to my friend Deborah, my little sister and I are huge fans of this recipe. Sometimes we like to have a slice for breakfast or dinner — it's that good!

GLUTEN-FREE PIE CRUST
>   3 cups gluten-free flour
>   1 teaspoon sea salt
>   ½ cup rice or almond milk, plus extra for brushing
>   ½ cup olive oil

FILLING
>   2 cans pumpkin puree
>   1 can organic coconut milk
>   ½ cup maple syrup
>   4 eggs
>   1 teaspoon sea salt
>   1 teaspoon each cinnamon, dried ginger, and allspice
>   1 teaspoon vanilla extract

Preheat oven to 350°F. To make the pie crust: Put the flour and salt in a food processor and pulse until mixed well. Put the milk and oil in a bowl and whisk together well. Add the liquid mixture to the flour as the food processor runs. Remove the dough and roll it out on wax paper to make an even, thin layer, about ⅛ inch thick. Cut the dough into two circles. Press one circle into a pie pan. To make the filling: Put all ingredients into a food processor and puree until well blended.

Pour the filling into the prepared pan and top with the second crust. Press the edges of the two crust layers together with a fork, and then trim the excess. Brush the top crust with milk, and then make slits in it to let out steam. Bake for about an hour or until the top crust is nicely browned and starts to crack.

> ### TRY THIS
>
> If you need to destress amid the workday's tensions or while winding down for sleep, sip some chamomile tea. If you like, sweeten it with some honey, agave, or stevia. This herb eases nervousness, anxiety, stress, and insomnia while improving immunity and soothing the digestive tract. *For pregnant women:* some herbalists have said this is too relaxing to the uterus to consume during pregnancy.

GRATITUDE

I was born on Thanksgiving — maybe that's why it's my favorite holiday. But I also love its significance. I appreciate how it's a day that anyone, anywhere, can celebrate, for it simply calls us to come together in community and say thank you. Gratitude is one of the most medicinal emotions we can feel. It elevates our moods and fills us with joy.

This season, not just on Thanksgiving, but at least at one meal a day, share a blessing of gratitude before you eat. Choose one of your own, or use this mealtime blessing from Vietnamese monk Thich Nhat Hanh:

1. *Serving food:* In this food I see clearly the presence of the entire universe supporting my existence.

2. *Looking at the filled plate:* All living beings are struggling for life. May they all have enough food to eat today.

3. *Just before eating:* The plate is filled with food. I am aware that each morsel is the fruit of much hard work by those who produced it.

4. *Beginning to eat:* With the first taste, I promise to practice loving-kindness. With the second, I promise to relieve the suffering of others. With the third, I promise to see others' joy as my own. With the fourth, I promise to learn the way of nonattachment and equanimity.

5. *Finishing the meal:* The plate is empty. My hunger is satisfied. I vow to live for the benefit of all beings.[2]

Taking a moment to give thanks before eating helps to restore the sacred balance that this planet needs to survive. Before our ancestors killed the animals that they would feast on, they offered prayers and rituals. The food you eat is a gift from the Great Mother so that you can share your own gifts with the world in the highest possible way.

DAILY GRATITUDE LIST

Make a nightly ritual of writing down all the things that you're grateful for from that day. If you sleep with your partner, share your lists with each other. Nothing's too insignificant to include here. You might be surprised at how much you appreciate the simplest things from your day (the way the light looked outside the window when you took a shower or the warm smile from a delivery person). A regular practice of this makes you more likely to honor these little gifts as they arise throughout your day.

Now we'll look at how to embody gratitude and the nurturance of autumn more deeply inside our bodies and hearts as we step onto our yoga mats.

REMEMBER

- Choose heavier, denser, cooked foods to ground and insulate you during the cold weather.
- Take special care of yourself this season. Doing so will help keep you healthy through the winter and beyond. Sleep more, be gentle, and get back into a routine.
- Delight in the fragrant dishes you create. Invite others to partake in the nourishment.
- Share a gratitude blessing before at least one meal each day — and as often as you can throughout the day. Gratitude is a major key to ongoing health and happiness!

Chapter 16

ON *the* YOGA MAT
Gathering Strength

It's really easy to get overstimulated in the fall: going back to school, gearing up for holiday festivities, grunting out that final push for the fourth quarter of the fiscal year. Amid it all, like faithful friends, your yoga and meditation practices await you. They serve as your refuge, offering a quiet space in which to ground yourself, clear your mind, and reconnect with what truly matters. This makes it easier to say no to the extraneous in order to say yes to what you truly desire. If you are in the process of letting go of something or someone, these practices will put you in touch with that which never changes — loving presence. With the slow yet dynamic practices for the fall season, you learn that it's okay to start slowing down and listening to your inner wisdom.

Since the sun starts rising later and later as this season progresses, it can become increasingly challenging to get up and moving in the early morning. However, if you're an early bird, go ahead! If you're feeling cold and sluggish, you can start with the yin practice in the morning to gently get your energy flowing again. Then you can do the flow practice later on in the afternoon when you're feeling more warmed up. The late morning, at least two hours after breakfast and right before lunch, can be a nice time to practice during these colder months too, if your schedule affords you that luxury.

Practice near a window to keep a connection with nature — especially amid the beautiful colors of leaves and light that are available during these months. For the flow practice, you can use a space heater or practice next to a fireplace or wood-burning stove to help get a sweat going and move toxins out through your skin.

OVERCOMING OVERWHELM

Anxiety can increase in the autumn amid all the outer and inner changes. Here are some tips for working with it skillfully:

1. Review your Absolute Yes and Absolute No Lists from chapter 5. Update them as necessary, and post them in a prominent place. Keep your boundaries clear and energy contained by really sticking to them this season.
2. When you feel overwhelm coming on, ask yourself, "What's most essential right now?" Then act from that place.
3. Give yourself permission to be spacious. Go for a long walk in the middle of the workday, take a nap, or read something relaxing. Trust that you'll actually get more done when you work from a place of relaxed ease rather than one of nervous stress.
4. Meditate on sounds. Take five or ten minutes to turn away from your thoughts and listen to your environment — the wind, the birds, the whiz of cars passing by. Tap into the underlying, patient hush that is always present and of which you too are a part (even when your mind's jumping around like a crazed monkey).
5. Ask yourself each day, What would taking really good care of myself look like right now?

EMOTIONAL AND MENTAL QUALITIES
OF THE LUNGS AND LARGE INTESTINE

Like the heart and small intestine, which though physically distant from each other are close energetic allies, the lungs and large intestine have a similar relationship, in that their alliance gives life to your whole being. Constantly drawing in nutrients and expelling wastes, they officiate how well (or how poorly) we assimilate the vital life force energy from the outside world and make it a part of who we are. They remind us that we always have everything we need — but the question is, How well do we receive it and then let go of the extraneous?

A healthy lung–large intestine system allows us to courageously feel the tenderness of life's fleeting moments without being crushed by them. Sometimes acknowledging the passing of beauty — whether in the form of a loved one leaving or of a simple sunset after a wonderful day — can elicit great and beautiful sadness. Living fully and passionately requires you to be a warrioress, to stand steady as both a participant in and a witness to the poignancy in each moment, always staying rooted in the wisdom and nobility of your heart. You have the strength to feel sadness and grief from deep loss, and you also have the resilience not to get buried under their heaviness for longer than you need to. Healthy lung and large intestine chi means that you fully accept life's continual invitation for us to dance with letting go.

AUTUMN YIN YOGA

By targeting the lung and large intestine meridians, this yin yoga sequence supports the release of emotions so that you can feel the sorrows of life as gateways to appreciating its preciousness. Taste and live them fully, with courage and gratitude, and then release your grip on them without excessive grief, sadness, or despair.

The lung meridian travels down to the large intestine from the core of the body and then loops up again through the diaphragm and lungs, and then down the underside of the arm to end at the tip of your thumb. Its partner meridian, that of the large intestine, starts at the index finger, journeys up to the shoulder, and then goes through the face to end at the side of the nose, while another branch descends through the lungs, diaphragm, and large intestine.

Before Beginning: Review the sections "Create a Sacred Space" (page 67) and "Yin Yoga" (page 49).

Intention: To release and let go amid life's changes while feeling everything deeply and courageously.

Total Practice Time: 60 minutes

Full Sequence of Illustrations: Page 212

1. *Check-In and Intention* (2 to 3 minutes): You can review these in chapter 3.
2. *Tree Visualization* (2 to 5 minutes): Stay sitting cross-legged on your mat. Close your eyes. Rest your palms on your midthighs to help you feel grounded and rooted like a tree. Imagine that from your belly button downward you are a tree trunk. Feel the roots in your pelvis stretching all the way down, deep into the dark soil of the earth. Envision and embody that for a few minutes.

    Stay with this visualization now as you inhale and focus on expanding the branches of the tree — let your chest fill as you breathe in. Breathe into the tops, bottoms, sides, fronts, and backs of your lungs. Then, as you

FALL YIN YOGA SEQUENCE

1. Check-In
and Intention

2. Tree
Visualization

3. Butterfly Pose

4. Saddle or Sphinx Pose

5. Sphinx Pose

6. Seal or Sphinx Pose

7. Seed Pose

8. One-Knee Spinal
Twist

9. Snail Pose

10. Fish Pose

11. Full Forward
Fold

12. Legs Up
the Wall Pose

13. Compassion
Meditation

14. Dedication
of Merit

exhale, draw your belly back to your spine. Feel an emptying in your lower body. Do that several times. Keep your inhalation and exhalation of equal lengths. Use this same breath concentration throughout the practice to enliven your lungs and soothe and ground your large intestine.

3. *Butterfly Pose* (5 minutes): See page 164.

4. *Saddle* or *Sphinx Pose* (5 minutes): From Butterfly Pose, swing your legs back behind you and sit on your heels. Make sure your big toes are touching and your knees are spread wide apart. Now slowly lean back and prop yourself up on your forearms. If that feels okay,

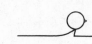

then you can lean all the way back onto the ground, your arms stretched out long behind you. *Note:* If you have any lower-back or knee pain, please play it safe and practice Sphinx or Seal Pose instead (see page 110).

To come out of Saddle Pose, prop yourself up on your forearms, engage your abdominals, and slowly come back up to sitting. Come into Child's Pose (see page 109) for 5 breaths. If you're in Sphinx Pose, lie down on your belly and turn your head to one side.

5. *Sphinx Pose* (5 minutes): See page 110. Afterward, lie down on your belly and turn your head to one side. Rest here for a few breaths.

6. *Seal* or *Sphinx Pose* (5 minutes): See page 110. Then lie down on your belly, and turn your head to the other side. Rest here for a few breaths. *Note:* In both Seal and Sphinx Poses, to further stimulate the lung and large intestine meridians, press down through your thumb (lung point) and your index finger (large intestine). After, come into Child's Pose for 5 breaths.

7. *Seed Pose* (5 minutes): Lie down on your back, and hug your knees to your chest. As much as you can, keep the back of your pelvis on the mat. Relax your feet. Tuck your chin slightly. Soften your shoulders toward the ground, and rest your hands on the tops of your shins.

8. *One-Knee Spinal Twist* (5 minutes on each side): See page 112. Twist to the right first. To come out, draw your knees to your chest in Seed Pose for a few breaths.

9. *Snail Pose* (5 minutes): From Seed Pose, rock your hips up so they rest in the palms of your hands with your elbows on the floor, propping up your hips. Swing your legs back over your head. If your feet touch the ground behind you, release your hands from under your hips and stretch them back behind you, or interlace your hands on the backs of your shins or ankles. *Note:* If you have any neck injuries or are menstruating, put your legs up the wall or come into Supine Butterfly Pose instead (see page 112). To come out, slowly roll down and draw your knees into your chest in Seed Pose.

10. *Fish Pose* (1 to 3 minutes): Lie down on your back and put the soles of your feet together, opening your knees out to the sides in a Supine Butterfly Pose. Place your

hands on the undersides of your thighs and, as you inhale, lift up your chest to rest the top of your head on the floor so that your back arches and your sternum puffs. Breathe deeply into your chest. To come down, exhale and tuck your chin into your chest and slowly roll back to the ground, gripping your thighs with your hands for support. Then rock up to sitting.

11. *Full Forward Fold* (5 minutes): See page 165.

12. *Legs Up the Wall Pose* (5 minutes): Scoot up next to a wall, with a blanket or mat underneath you. Swing your legs up so there's a 90-degree angle between your legs and torso. If that feels like too much of a strain on your lower back or the backs of your legs, scoot your hips farther away from the wall. Rest your arms out to the sides, palms facing up. If you're menstruating, practice Supine Butterfly Pose instead (page 112). Close your eyes.

13. *Joy Meditation* (5 to 30 minutes): Cross your legs (the other leg on top now), and follow the meditation instructions on page 226.

14. *Dedication of Merit* (1 minute): Please review instructions on page 52.

MINI-AUTUMN YIN PRACTICE

Short on time? String these three poses together for a twenty-minute practice. Try them during your lunch break, as your child naps, before your morning shower, or just before sleep.

1. Butterfly Pose
2. Saddle Pose (or Sphinx Pose)
3. One-Knee Spinal Twist (both sides; complete this with a few breaths in Seed Pose)

AUTUMN FLOW YOGA

As you start spending more time inside this season (and savoring richer, denser foods), it's a good idea to stay active. This sets the pace through the wintertime so you don't get too stationary. Also, with all the changes this season, you can be more prone to spaciness, scattered thinking, and feeling disconnected from yourself and others. This practice builds mental clarity and focus, as well as physical grounding. Emotionally, this dynamic yoga sequence will empower you to face difficulties with verve, poise, confidence, and perseverance. While a little wallowing is a good thing, too much of it will snuff your inner spark. Part of the following sequence is inspired by the Ashtanga vinyasa tradition. It's great for building heat, strength, and a strong internal focus.

Before Beginning: Review the sections "Create a Sacred Space" (page 67) and "Yang (or Flow) Yoga" (page 50).

Intention: To build physical strength in your legs and a sense of rooting and grounding while garnering a mental clarity and emotional tenacity.

Total Practice Time: 60 minutes

Full Sequence of Illustrations: Pages 216–19

1. *Check-In and Intention* (2 to 5 minutes): Please revisit chapter 3 for details.
2. *Victorious Breath with Three-Part Breath* (3 minutes): While seated, combine the sound and quality of Victorious Breath (page 113) and stretch it out into the three-part breath to fill your belly, solar plexus, chest, neck, and head (page 166).
3. *Cat/Cow Pose* (5 to 10 rounds): See page 118.
4. *Lateral Cat/Cow Pose* (3 rounds): From your hands and knees, swing your hips to your right, looking over your right shoulder to compress your right waist. Then repeat on the left.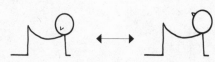
5. *Downward-Facing Dog* (5 breaths): Exhale into it. See page 118.
6. *Standing Forward Fold* (3 breaths): Walk your feet forward so they're hip width apart between your hands. See page 118.
7. *Chi Generation* (3 minutes): From the forward bend, bring your hands to your hips and inhale up to standing. Now take your feet a little wider than hip width and keep their outer edges parallel. Bend your knees deeply, and lift your arms up so they form a circle out in front of you, as if you're hugging a big tree. Keep your tailbone pointed down toward the floor and your spine vertical. Breathe deeply, and keep softening into the sensation. Spread and relax your feet as you root

AUTUMN FLOW YOGA SEQUENCE

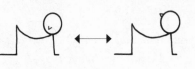

1. Check-In
and Intention

2. Victorious Breath
with Three-Part Breath

3. Cat Pose

Cow Pose

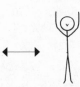

4. Lateral Cow Pose

5. Downward-Facing
Dog

6. Standing
Forward Fold

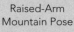

7. Chi Generation

8. Mountain Pose

9. Mountain Pose Toe Lifts

**10. ½ Sun
Salutation A
*(3 rounds)***

Mountain Pose

Raised-Arm
Mountain Pose

Standing Forward
Fold

½ Standing
Forward Fold

Standing Forward
Fold

Raised-Arm
Mountain Pose

**11. Sun
Salutation A
*(3 rounds)***

Mountain Pose

Raised-Arm
Mountain Pose

Standing Forward
Fold

AUTUMN FLOW YOGA SEQUENCE (CONTINUED)

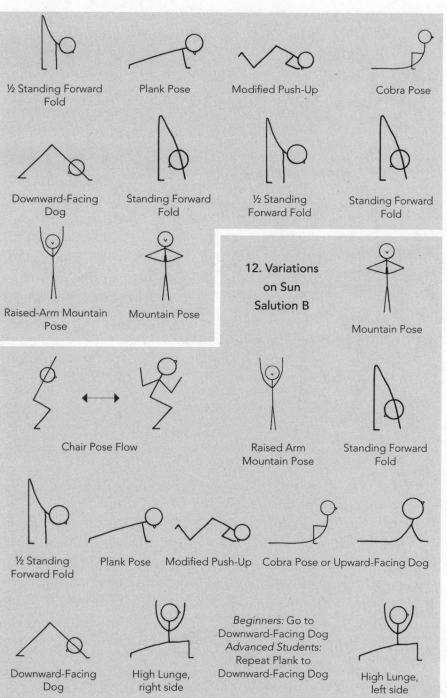

½ Standing Forward Fold

Plank Pose

Modified Push-Up

Cobra Pose

Downward-Facing Dog

Standing Forward Fold

½ Standing Forward Fold

Standing Forward Fold

Raised-Arm Mountain Pose

Mountain Pose

12. Variations on Sun Salution B

Mountain Pose

Chair Pose Flow

Raised Arm Mountain Pose

Standing Forward Fold

½ Standing Forward Fold

Plank Pose

Modified Push-Up

Cobra Pose or Upward-Facing Dog

Downward-Facing Dog

High Lunge, right side

Beginners: Go to Downward-Facing Dog
Advanced Students: Repeat Plank to Downward-Facing Dog

High Lunge, left side

AUTUMN FLOW YOGA SEQUENCE (CONTINUED)

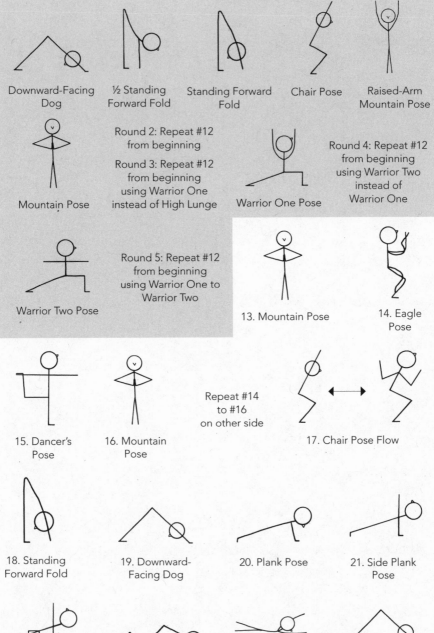

Downward-Facing Dog

½ Standing Forward Fold

Standing Forward Fold

Chair Pose

Raised-Arm Mountain Pose

Mountain Pose

Round 2: Repeat #12 from beginning

Round 3: Repeat #12 from beginning using Warrior One instead of High Lunge

Warrior One Pose

Round 4: Repeat #12 from beginning using Warrior Two instead of Warrior One

Warrior Two Pose

Round 5: Repeat #12 from beginning using Warrior One to Warrior Two

13. Mountain Pose

14. Eagle Pose

15. Dancer's Pose

16. Mountain Pose

Repeat #14 to #16 on other side

17. Chair Pose Flow

18. Standing Forward Fold

19. Downward-Facing Dog

20. Plank Pose

21. Side Plank Pose

Side Plank Pose for Beginners

22. Modified Push-Up

23. Alternating Locust Pose

24. Downward-Facing Dog

AUTUMN FLOW YOGA SEQUENCE *(CONTINUED)*

25. Standing
Forward Fold

26. Chair Pose

27. Raised-Arm
Mountain Pose

28. Mountain Pose

29. Repeat #16 to #23
on other side

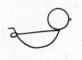

30. Bow Pose

31. Downward-
Facing Dog

32. Child's Pose

33. Headstand

34. Child's Pose

35. Downward-
Facing Dog

36. Staff Pose

37. Shoelace Pose

38. Staff Pose

39. One-Leg Seated
Spinal Twist

40. One-Leg Seated
Forward Fold

41. Lateral One-Leg
Seated Forward Fold

42. Repeat #37 to #41
on other side

43. Butterfly Pose

44. Final Relaxation
Pose

45. Bumblebee Breath

46. Joy
Meditation

47. Dedication of Merit

your legs down into the earth. Bend your knees as deeply as you can, and embrace any discomfort with your deep breaths.

8. *Mountain Pose* (5 breaths): See page 119.

9. *Mountain Pose Toe Lifts* (5 rounds): From Mountain Pose, exhale and release your hands down. Inhale and sweep your arms out to your sides and all the way overhead as you lift up onto your tiptoes. Exhale and release your arms down by your sides again as you lower your heels to the ground. Repeat four more times, and on your fifth round, stay up on your tiptoes for five breaths before lowering down.

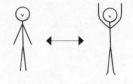

10. *½ Sun Salutation A*
    - *Mountain Pose:* Exhale into it.
    - *Raised-Arm Mountain Pose:* Inhale into it. See page 171.
    - *Standing Forward Fold:* Exhale into it.
    - *½ Standing Forward Fold:* Inhale into it. See page 170.
    - *Standing Forward Fold:* Exhale into it.
    - *Raised-Arm Mountain Pose:* Inhale into it.
    - Repeat 2 more times.

11. *Sun Salutation A*
    - *Mountain Pose:* Exhale into it.
    - *Raised-Arm Mountain Pose:* Inhale into it.
    - *Standing Forward Fold:* Exhale into it.
    - *½ Standing Forward Fold:* Inhale into it.
    - *Plank Pose:* Step or jump back to this pose as you exhale. See page 120.
    - *Modified Push-Up:* Exhale into it. See page 171.
    - *Cobra Pose:* On your belly, place your hands under your shoulders, inhale and lift your chest, keeping your hips rooted, elbows bent, and legs outstretched behind you.
    - *Downward-Facing Dog* (5 breaths): Come into it on an exhale. See instructions on page 118.
    - *Standing Forward Fold:* Step or jump into it as you exhale.
    - *½ Standing Forward Fold:* Inhale into it.
    - *Standing Forward Fold:* Exhale into it.
    - *Raised-Arm Mountain Pose:* Inhale into it.
    - *Mountain Pose:* Exhale into it.
    - Repeat 2 more times.

12. *Variations on Sun Salutation B*
  - *Mountain Pose* (5 breaths).
  - *Chair Pose Flow* (5 rounds): Exhale into 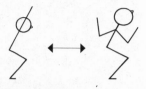 Chair Pose, and then on the inhale, stay in it as you lift your arms overhead. Exhale, and keep your knees bent as you bend your elbows in toward your side ribs and look up. Inhale, and keep your knees bent, deepening here if you can as you straighten your arms overhead and look down toward your feet. Repeat four more times.
  - *Raised-Arm Mountain Pose:* Inhale into it.
  - *Standing Forward Fold* (5 breaths): Exhale into it, and hold.
  - *½ Standing Forward Fold:* Inhale into it.
  - *Plank Pose* (5 breaths): Step or jump into it as you exhale, and hold.
  - *Modified Push-Up:* Exhale into it.
  - *Cobra Pose* or *Upward-Facing Dog* (5 breaths): For Upward-Facing Dog, place your hands on the mat directly under your shoulders. Inhale and lift your chest and hips off the floor, rolling your shoulders back, keeping elbows softly bent and pressing tops of feet into the mat. Inhale, and hold.
  - *Downward-Facing Dog* (5 breaths): Exhale, and hold.
  - *High Lunge* (5 breaths): Inhale, and step your right foot forward (see page 121).
  - *Beginners:* Go straight to Downward-Facing Dog. *Advanced students:* Go to Plank Pose, Push-Up, Cobra or Upward-Facing Dog, and Downward-Facing Dog.
  - *High Lunge* (5 breaths): Left foot forward. Repeat the instructions above for beginners and advanced students.
  - *Downward-Facing Dog* (5 breaths).
  - *½ Standing Forward Fold:* Step or jump forward as you exhale, then inhale into it.
  - *Standing Forward Fold* (5 breaths): Exhale into it.
  - *Chair Pose* (5 breaths): Inhale into it.
  - *Raised-Arm Mountain Pose:* Inhale into it.
  - *Mountain Pose:* Exhale, and hold for 5 breaths.
  - Repeat the above sequence again with High Lunge. For the third round, instead of the High Lunge, turn the back foot out slightly and place it fully on the ground. Come up into Warrior One Position. Square your hips forward with your front thigh parallel to the floor and

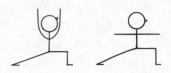

your front knee over your front ankle. Stretch your arms up next to your ears. Hold for 5 breaths in Warrior One on each side. For the fourth round, replace Warrior One with Warrior Two (see page 121). For the fifth and final round, move from Warrior One to Warrior Two, and hold each for 5 breaths.

13. *Mountain Pose:* Pause for 5 to 10 breaths, letting your inhalations and exhalations even and lengthen out — about 5 counts for the in-breath and 5 counts for the out-breath.

14. *Eagle Pose* (5 breaths): Shift your weight onto your right foot. Lift your left foot off the ground, and cross your left knee over your right, as if you're sitting with your legs crossed in an invisible chair. If you can, tuck your left toes behind your right calf. Then inhale and swing your arms out into a T position. As you exhale, cross your left elbow under your right, then cross at your wrists so your palms press into each other. Lower your sitting bones close to your heels as you stay buoyant in your chest. Slide your shoulder blades down your back as you reach up to the sky with your fingertips. *Beginners:* You can hold on to a wall here. Just cross your left knee over your right, and don't worry about tucking the foot behind or crossing your arms.

15. *Dancer's Pose:* From Eagle Pose, unwrap your arms and your left leg. Take hold of the outside edge of your left foot with your left hand behind you, so that your heel is in close to your left buttock. Stretch your right arm straight out in front of you at shoulder height. Press your left leg back into your hand, eventually kicking the foot up to the height of your head behind you. Keep squaring your hips and shoulders to the front of the room, staying tall and open through your torso. Hold here for 5 breaths. *Beginners:* Stay with your left heel close to your buttock. Hold on to a wall if you need more support.

16. *Mountain Pose:* Return here and then repeat Eagle Pose and Dancer's Pose on the other side. Return to Mountain Pose after the second side.

17. *Chair Pose Flow* (5 rounds): Exhale into it.

18. *Standing Forward Fold* (5 breaths): Exhale into it.

19. *Downward-Facing Dog* (5 breaths): Exhale into it.

20. *High Plank Pose* (5 breaths): Inhale into it.

21. *Side Plank Pose* (5 breaths on each side): Shift your weight onto your right hand, and stack your left foot on top of your right. Stretch your left arm up to the sky, and keep lifting your hips away from the mat. Then repeat on the other side, pausing in between in Downward-Facing Dog or Child's Pose if you need to. *Beginners:* Place your top foot down on the floor in front of you, with the knee bent for more support.

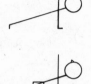

22. *Modified Push-Up* (5 breaths): Lower down to the ground slowly.

23. *Alternating Locust Pose* (5 rounds): On your belly, stretch your arms straight out in front of you, forehead on the mat. Inhale and lift your chest, left leg, and right arm, bringing the arm next to your ear. Exhale and lower down, and then repeat on the other side. Do this 4 times, and on the fifth time, hold in the up position on each side for 5 breaths.

24. *Downward-Facing Dog* (5 breaths): Exhale into it.

25. *Standing Forward Fold* (5 breaths): Exhale into it.

26. *Chair Pose* (5 breaths): Inhale into it.

27. *Raised-Arm Mountain Pose:* Inhale into it.

28. *Mountain Pose* (5 breaths): Exhale into it.

29. Repeat 16 to 23 on the other side.

30. *Bow Pose:* From Alternating Locust Pose, reach back and hold the outside of each foot with your hands. As you inhale, press your feet back into your hands and lift your chest. Reach your inner heels up to the ceiling as you balance on your pubic bone. *Tip:* If this feels uncomfortable, place a blanket underneath you for this pose. Beginners can put a strap around each ankle to help reach the feet. Hold for 5 to 10 breaths. Lower down slowly, and rest on your belly for 5 to 10 breaths.

31. *Downward-Facing Dog* (5 breaths): Exhale into it.

32. *Child's Pose* (5 breaths): Exhale into it.

33. *Headstand* (10 to 30 breaths): If you're new to headstands, I suggest you learn this with a teacher to make sure that you have the correct alignment. If you're menstruating or have a headache, do Legs Up the Wall for a few minutes instead (see page 214).

34. *Child's Pose* (5 breaths): Exhale into it.

35. *Downward-Facing Dog* (5 breaths): Exhale into it.

36. *Staff Pose:* Come to a seated posture, with your legs stretched out in front of you, feet outer hip width apart. Place your fingertips behind you, and lift and broaden your chest. Breathe deeply into your heart and lungs for 5 breaths while feeling your legs and pelvis firmly rooted on the ground.

37. *Shoelace Pose* (5 breaths on each side): From Staff Pose, bend your right leg and stack your right knee on top of your left. Stay there, or to go further, bend your left knee as well. This is the same position as Shoelace Pose in chapter 8's yin sequence (see page 110). Stay upright for 5 breaths, and then fold forward for 5 more. Inhale to come up, and repeat on the other side.

38. *Staff Pose* (5 breaths).

39. *One-Leg Seated Spinal Twist:* Draw your right heel in; place it just to the outside of your left knee. Place your right hand behind your right hip, raised up on the fingertips. Inhale, and lift your left arm. Exhale, and place your left elbow outside your right knee. Gently twist over to the right, looking over your right shoulder. *Beginners:* You can wrap your left arm around your right knee instead of hooking the elbow outside the knee.

40. *One-Leg Seated Forward Fold* (5 breaths): Exhale and return to center. Inhale as you bring your right foot to the inside of your left thigh and open your right knee out to the side. Bring your right heel to the very top of your left thigh. Square your hips and shoulders over your left leg. Inhale and lengthen your spine. Exhale and fold forward over your left leg. *Beginners:* You can bring the sole of your right foot to the inside of your left thigh. Place a blanket under your right thigh if you need more support for your right knee. Inhale and slowly rise.

41. *Lateral One-Leg Seated Forward Fold* (5 breaths): Open your right knee a bit farther out to the right and turn your belly so it's aiming to the space in between your right knee and left toes. Take your left elbow to the floor or a block in front of your left knee. Inhale and lift your right arm up. If you can go farther, stretch it over your head, eventually taking hold of your left foot. Keep your chest open, twisting up toward the ceiling.

42. Repeat 37 to 41 on the other side.

43. *Butterfly Pose:* Bring the soles of your feet together. Inhale and lengthen your spine. Exhale and extend forward. When you've come as far forward as you can, round your spine evenly over your bent legs, keeping your pelvis rooted. Stay here for 5 to 10 breaths. *Beginners:* Place a cushion or blankets underneath your knees for support if you need to. Stay upright for 5 full breaths.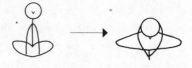

44. *Final Relaxation Pose* (5 to 10 minutes): See page 126.

45. *Bumblebee Breath* (5 minutes): Come to a comfortable seated posture. Close your eyes. Place your thumbs over your ears, closing you off from sound. Place your index fingers over your eyelids, closing you off from sight. Place your middle fingers gently over the nostrils (don't close yourself off from breath yet); and place your ring and pinky fingers over your mouth. Inhale through both nostrils, then close them with your middle fingers. As you exhale, keep your mouth closed and make a buzzing sound, like a bumblebee. Exhale for as long as you can. Repeat this for 1 to 5 minutes, being soothed by the sound of your own breath. When breath and sound come together like this, it relieves anxiety and excessive mental activity, dropping you into a deeper sense of inner peace.

46. *Joy Meditation* (5 to 30 minutes): Read the instructions on the next page.

47. *Dedication of Merit* (1 minute): Please review instructions on page 52.

MINI-AUTUMN FLOW PRACTICE

If you're short on time, you can do this one in fifteen to twenty minutes:

1. Cat/Cow (5 rounds)
2. Chi Generation (3 minutes)
3. ½ Sun Salutation A (twice)
4. Sun Salutation A (twice)
5. Variations on Sun Salutation B (1 round with High Lunge, second round with Warrior One, third round with Warrior Two)
6. One-Leg Seated Forward Fold (both sides)
7. Butterfly Pose
8. Final Relaxation (2 to 3 minutes)

JOY MEDITATION

My older sister and her husband spent a year trying to get pregnant (they now have two beautiful boys). During that time many of my sister's friends were getting pregnant effortlessly. And it seemed that every time she stepped out onto the Chicago streets, she saw new mothers happily pushing their new babies around town in their strollers. She was trying to balance her despair of having another negative pregnancy test with the joy she should feel after getting a voice mail from a friend announcing her pregnancy.

> ### TRY THIS
>
> Give some extra TLC to your lungs this season by consciously taking deep breaths. Make it fun: instead of tensing up and spiraling into negativity and worry whenever you get a stressful email or phone call, take a full breath instead. Expand your rib cage as wide as you can with the breath; fill it as if it were an umbrella opening out in all directions. Even better, take little breaks outside during your day to soak up some sun, and breathe in the fresh, autumn air. Just as your digestive system thrives from the nutrients it extracts from healthy foods, your lungs appreciate the vital life force in fresh air.

"I feel jealous and happy for her at the same time. A part of me can't help but think, 'It's not fair.' I want that to be me," she shared with honest vulnerability.

We've all been there. If you just got dumped and a friend scored a handsome and loving husband, can you separate the two occurrences without needing to compare them? If another friend has been working out a lot and is looking strong and energized while you've been slaving away like a madwoman on your business, be inspired by her physique rather than jealous of it. I'm not saying that you should deny what you feel. Feel the jealousy, the anger, your own perceived sense of lack. Feel it fully, and then ask yourself if that's really how you want to respond. Is there another, more skillful and connecting response that you can choose? Each person gets exactly what she needs to grow into her greatest self. When you see life this way, there's no longer a need to compare or compete. Every situation is an opportunity to grow.

In Buddhism, this quality is known as "sympathetic joy." It simply means being able to feel joy at the good fortune of others.[1]

Once you genuinely feel excited for friends, you can then extend these blessings to neutral people, to enemies, and eventually to all beings (including yourself). Also, the more you allow yourself to feel your sadness as it arises, the more you grow your capacity to also experience joy. Here's how to do it:

1. Begin with Mindfulness Meditation for at least five minutes. (See page 44.)
2. Picture in your mind's eye the person whom you wish to be happy. Say these words to her or him, by repeating them silently to yourself:

May you be filled with joy.
May your joy, happiness, and good fortune increase.
May you always live in alignment with your greatest happiness.
May the causes of your joy, happiness, and good fortune continue to grow.

Whenever your mind wanders, bring it back to these words. Continue on, no matter what feelings come up. Stay with it. Do this for about five minutes.

3. Return to Mindfulness Meditation for another minute, and then bow gently to yourself and to the spirit of your friend who came to teach you how to choose supportiveness over competition.

Let's journey deeper now into your spirit to see what you have learned throughout this season. Now's the time to decide: What are you leaving behind, and what are you taking with you into the dark winter months?

REMEMBER

- Return to your good friends — your yoga and meditation practices — to keep you grounded and sane during the hustle and bustle of going back to school or work.
- Practice yin yoga to find the inner spaciousness you need to let go, feel your feelings, and grieve for what you've lost.
- Build stability in your body and clarity in your mind through flow yoga.
- Celebrate the good fortune of others by cultivating sympathetic joy. Your neighbor got a shiny new car, and yours just went in the shop for the second time this month. Great! Another opportunity to practice...

Chapter 17

AUTUMN REFLECTIONS

The fleetingness of our precious lives feels more pronounced this season. All around us we see nature coming into ecstatic beauty and then, a day or two later, crumbling and withering. Leaves turn crimson and gold. Their luster fades as they dry and flutter to the ground, returning once again to the earth's soil. We say good-bye to the lightheartedness of summer and prepare to face the dark, quiet winter months ahead.

HONORING YOUR ANCESTORS

This is a powerful time to reflect on what really matters to you and to honor your ancestors, who paved the way for you to be here. Can you feel how you are standing on the shoulders of all the women who came before you? If you have pictures of them, take them out. Light candles for them. Place a flower in a vase near the photos. Visit them at the cemetery. Prepare ancestral foods such as your grandmother's famous lasagna or whatever recipes you pass on in your family. Ask your ancestors for their wisdom. Especially in Asian cultures, this is the acknowledged time of year when the presence of ancestors is the strongest, and you can access it through your prayer. Take out your journal and write about unresolved emotional pain and family wounds. Call on your ancestors for guidance and protection. Tell your children stories about your lineage, ask your parents about their childhoods, record oral history interviews with your relatives to pass on to future generations. There's an African proverb that says when an old man or woman dies, a library dies with him or her. Keep the chain of wisdom alive. We are all connected in an intricate, intimate web. The more we remember our place in this — and that we're not isolated entities — the stronger we will be.

Now, looking back over the past few months, take an honest look at how things have been for you, in both your outer and inner worlds, and explore them in your journal through the questions below.

MONTH ONE

1. At the start of this season, I felt most overwhelmed by and anxious about:
2. My main health concerns were:
3. The three main things that I know I need to let go of are:
4. The two ways I've enjoyed starting to slow down more are:
5. The one habit I'm going to focus on cultivating for the next thirty days is _____. I will omit _____ in order to create space for this. The three main things I hope to experience as a result of this are:

MONTH TWO

1. In looking back to the spring, what I'm harvesting in my life right now from those efforts are _____ and _____. The results I'm feeling are mostly _____ and _____.
2. The five main things that I'm wanting to bring with me into the rest of the year are:
3. I'm finding it hard to be happy for _____ because _____, but one way I can celebrate her or him is by _____.
4. Three things I'm feeling really grateful for are:
5. When I feel anxious and ungrounded, I usually feel it in my body the most in _____. When I feel rested and at ease, I usually feel it in my body as _____.

MONTH THREE

1. The things I'm celebrating most from my efforts this season are:
2. Looking back, I realize that my biggest challenges were:
3. The ancestors I feel most connected to are:
4. Their qualities and traditions that I want to keep alive in my life and my family are:
5. I omit my usual time wasters of _____ and _____ in order to make more quiet time for myself, which I want to spend by _____.

COMMUNITY RITUAL

This autumn I went to a Native American tipi ceremony one evening just as the temperature was starting to drop, marking the end of summer and the arrival of fall. Many members of my community and I sat around the fire to pray. Into the flames I spoke all those things I wanted to let go of and what I wanted to take with me on my life journey. I left feeling strong, grounded, and clear.

Group bonfires happen everywhere this season because they help us in our journey of letting go and transitioning into the darkest, coldest time of the year. As part of the Celtic Samhain, or "summer's end" tradition (which falls on the same day as Halloween in the United States), community members gather around a large bonfire. Come together around this ancient light to pray. Look into the flames and ask for support with your inner alchemy, the transformation of letting go. If you have physical things (old letters or photographs) that would symbolically help you to release the past, offer those to the fire too. These rituals take on a whole new depth when you do them in the loving presence of other people in your community — whether you include a few close friends or a much larger group. These gatherings have been lost in our modern culture, which values independence and isolation. But as tribal beings, we carry the memory of them in our DNA, and we still need these rituals for our health and healing.

From the reduction of autumn and the deep courage that's bolstered through the process of letting go, we'll journey as mystical warrioresses into the dreamtime of winter, carrying with us only what we need...

PART 5

WINTER

Element: WATER

Colors: BLUE AND BLACK

Organs: KIDNEYS AND BLADDER

Heart qualities: FEAR, WISDOM, AND EQUANIMITY

Life cycle: LATE ADULTHOOD

Creative cycle: DEATH, DESTRUCTION, AND VISIONING

Menstrual cycle: MENSTRUATION

Moon cycle: NEW MOON

Actions: REST, REFLECTION, AND PREPARATION

Focus: SOURCE YOUR INTUITION, INNER WISDOM, INDIGENOUS POWER, AND CREATIVE POTENTIAL THROUGH DEEP REST.

Chapter 18

LISTENING

In September 2001 I spent three weeks in Nepal. One
misty morning after a hearty breakfast of *tsampa* (a traditional Tibetan
porridge made from roasted barley flour) in the village inn, my guides, friend,
and I continued our trek, which we were already a few days into, along the An-
napurna Circuit. One of the guides had eaten breakfast in a separate room of
the inn, listening to the radio. As we began our walk later that morning, packs
on our backs, he reported, "A plane crashed into the World Trade Center in
New York City and also into the Pentagon in Washington, DC."

My family lived in New York City. My friend's family lived in Washington. Fear, anger, confusion, sadness, and grief washed through us both. There
was no way for our families to get in touch with us, and the next village, Marpa,
where we would spend that night — and where I hoped we could make a phone
call home and catch the news — was still several hours away. When we finally arrived in Marpa, Nepali villagers and international trekkers sat in shock
around the TV watching CNN. I managed to call home for a few minutes from
a pay phone, long enough to find out that everyone was okay.

At the end of the trip, I spent my final nights in Kathmandu before catching
a flight back to Bangkok. On my last morning there I woke up early and visited
the "monkey temple," Swayambhunath Stupa. Ever since I was a little girl, I
have had a strange longing to see a cremation, and that day I finally did. I sat on
the stone steps of the temple, watching the ritual of bodies burning — tended
to by prayer, song, incense, and seemingly choreographed movement by the
cremation attendants. The ash in the wind and the distinct smell of human flesh
aflame caused the hair on my body to stand on end. I was riveted. Here, the
body wasn't hidden in a casket or pumped up with formaldehyde and painted
with makeup. It was out in the daylight, raw and real, for everyone to see. The

several hours that the body took to burn allowed everyone present to see life return to ash. Those hours that I sat on the stone steps stand side by side in my memory with the fateful day of 9/11.

When we let it, death and destruction can bring us much closer together as human beings. We remember our vulnerability and the preciousness of being alive. We remember that we need one another and that we never know when death will come for us. We need to partake in the full ritual of death — however gritty it may be to witness — and the ensuing descent into the darkness of our own souls in order to sing loud and clear when the dawn comes again.

In the yearly cycle it's winter, in the daily cycle it's nighttime, and in the monthly cycle it's the new moon and menstruation that give us the opportunity to practice dying. However, these little deaths that compel us to grope through the dark nights of our souls are what most of us avoid the most. We'd rather just take a pill and be happy all the time than feel the searing pain of loss and of being lost. But there's a huge folly here. If we don't surrender and let things die away and dissolve into mystery and darkness, there's no space from which anything new can be reborn.

How can we rest in the stark stillness of the season without grasping for a plan or rushing on to the next big thing?

Winter, while it can be one of the hardest seasons to embrace, has a lot to teach us about true beauty and wisdom. Stripped of her flowers, leaves, and warmth, the earth reveals her naked self through her skeleton branches and barren ground. She becomes completely simple, having discarded everything but the bare essentials. Her scarcity and fierceness command our respect and attention, and, without apology for not being a warm and gracious hostess, she retreats into frozen silence. When we look to nature as our teacher, we see that she's reflecting back to us a prolonged opportunity to hibernate and renew. Arriving with the shortest day of the year on the winter solstice, December 21 (June 21 in the southern hemisphere), winter slowly grows brighter from this day on as the sun's presence gradually beams stronger and stronger until its apex on the next summer solstice. Hanukkah, Advent, Christmas, and Kwanza, along with many other holidays and rituals, celebrate the return of this light. We're reminded to connect with the sun within us, which is the bright potential of our souls, even amid the darkness and the holiday frenzy. We also celebrate

New Year's, a call to reflect on the past, appreciate the present, and dream our future. This truly is the time of year to go inside and ripen in our womanly wisdom before stepping out into the world again.

RECLAIMING REST

Use the darkness all around you to explore your inner world. There you will find that flame inside you that can never be extinguished. You can only make this descent when you commit to stillness, solitude, and deep soul-searching. You must become quiet, less social, more introverted, and — despite the negative connotations in most cultures — lazy. Just as fields need to remain fallow at times for their soil to stay fertile, we need to leave our innermost beings barren of new projects, adventures, and activities. We've done this in smaller doses during menstruation and the new moon, but this is downtime in a much bigger sense.

If we don't take time each year for deep rest, then authentic healing, rejuvenation, wisdom, and softening are not possible. It takes so much energy to burst forth into the world and to birth something new. This winter, treat yourself like a pregnant mama. Rest, nurture yourself, rebuild your vital life force, and prepare for the coming of new life. And if you don't live in an area with a pronounced winter season, you need to be more disciplined about getting quiet. This is also an opportunity to listen to the subtler rhythms of nature.

Yet while nature's saying one thing, society's saying another. We need to acknowledge that there is a reason why winter's wisdom is ignored in modern society. We've come to see rest as lazy and unproductive and have fallen in love with constant, linear progress. Saturdays, Sundays, and holidays are designated off days, and at all other times we're expected to be on. Within the cycle of life, late adulthood isn't valued either. Our elders are hidden away in old-age homes, no longer able to enrich the youth with their wisdom. There's a sad ignorance in this, a forgetting of how to honor the sacred balance by holding in equal esteem *all* of life's stages.

You, I know, are here because you've seen the fallacy in this denial of the dark, quiet point in the circle. You've seen how destructive it is for your health and happiness as a woman — as well as for your family and community. But we haven't just thumbed our noses at winter repose because of our prejudices about becoming soft and rested; we have also done this because we're afraid to face our own shadow sides. We're afraid of uncertainty. We don't want to look our sadness, our anger, or our fear in the eye and really ask what each has to teach us. When we avoid facing these less savory parts of ourselves, we're missing out on the opportunity to become who we truly are. Yes, it's messy. Yes, it feels uncomfortable. But by going to those depths you call in the light. You heal the parts of yourself that you have never wanted to acknowledge, much less learn to love. You must become the loving mother who calls all her lost children, or the estranged parts of yourself, home.

WOMB WISDOM

This wisdom I'm speaking of is a sort of deep knowing and indigenous power that perhaps you didn't even know you had. Yet *every* woman has it; it's called womb wisdom. This earthy, instinctual knowing of life's deepest truths lives in your uterus (even energetically, if you no longer have one physically), which you can also begin to think of as your second heart. The voice of your intuition comes from your womb. She has spoken to women and guided them through life's sometimes soft and sometimes vicious cycles of birth, blooming, death, and rebirth for millennia. She's here speaking to you now too. Winter, as well as your moon time, is when you can strengthen your alliance with her.

In addition to being deeply sensitive and emotional, your womb (as well as your ovaries) is your creative space — literally, in that this is the space where a baby comes into being, and metaphorically as well. From here you might launch a new career, make a collage, or write a book. When your womb is shut down energetically, your creativity is quashed. You might eventually experience this at the physical level through infertility or other gynecological complications, such as fibroids, cysts, or irregular cycles. To remedy a disconnection from your womb wisdom, you must first reclaim the artist that you are. Perhaps you've never thought of yourself as such, but now you need to start owning your creative genius. Your creativity comes through when you cook a meal, dress your daughter, decide what shoes to wear, and create a home. The more you take pause in your life, the more room there is for your inspiration to emerge within you.

I believe with (both) my hearts that *every* woman needs to strengthen her connection with her womb and support it in any way she can. This space harbors our deepest dreams and desires, as well as our capacity for nurturing ourselves and all beings. When we heal our relationships to our wombs and their wisdom we play a tremendous role in reviving for the world the lost qualities of creativity, intuition, feminine wisdom, and cyclical living.

TRY THIS

An Ayurvedic ritual for strengthening your womb energy as prescribed by Maya Tiwari involves the use of a hot ginger compress. Ginger, which you'll learn more about in the next chapter, is one of the best herbs to use this season because of its warming qualities. Keep in mind that it's best to do this ritual when you're not menstruating (since your body is already producing a lot of heat). At other times of the month, this compress can help to alleviate lower-back pain and energize the kidneys if you're feeling run-down. The ginger's warmth stimulates circulation and nourishes the downward-flowing energy in the body that governs elimination and menstruation. It's best to recruit a friend, daughter, or spouse to help you out with this, but you can also do it for yourself if you need to.

To make the compress, bring a gallon of water to a boil in a large stainless-steel pot. Juice a handful of freshly grated ginger, adding the juice to the water. If you don't have a juicer, put the grated ginger in a cloth tea bag or tie it into a piece of cheesecloth. Firmly squeeze the bag over the water, and then drop the whole bag into the pot. Reduce the heat and let the ginger water simmer for 30 minutes.

While that's simmering, set up some blankets on the floor and have a hand towel nearby. Remove the pot from the heat, and let it sit for 5 minutes. Rub warm sesame oil into your lower back. Then, before lying down, take the hand towel, holding both ends of it, and dip it into the pot of ginger water. Twist out the excess water. Cover the pot so that the contents stay hot. Test the temperature of the towel on your arm. When it is a comfortable temperature, fold the towel and place it directly over the kidney area of your lower back (just under your lowest ribs). You can keep your hand on it to provide pressure.

Stay here for 5 to 10 minutes, resting and breathing deeply. Repeat this 3 to 5 more times. At the end of your treatment, once again rub warm sesame oil into your lower back, and savor the feeling of warmth through your lower belly and lower back.[1]

WINTER RETREAT

THE ONE-DAY WINTER REJUVENATION RETREAT

Winter's the season most conducive to retreating. I sat my first thirty-day meditation retreat in Chiang Mai during the monsoon season, and it's much easier to stay inside and do your practice when the sun isn't shining and people aren't out playing. Use this day to embody all the practices outlined for this season and, most important, to rest. You might find it helpful to do it the week between Christmas and New Year's to recharge your batteries. Remember to completely unplug today: turn off your phone and computer, and enjoy a day of silence. The night before, soak the beans for the Three-Bean Chili (recipe on page 254), which you'll be having for lunch!

- Let yourself sleep as long as you need to.
- Before you get out of bed, write down your dreams in your journal (see page 242), in as much detail as you can.
- Set the intention to observe your thoughts throughout the day and to avoid complaining. Our thoughts become things. Since you are deep in your visionary stage, ask yourself what thoughts you are nurturing to become your reality.
- Scrape your tongue, brush your teeth, and use your neti pot.
- Drink one or two glasses of warm water with lemon, followed by a cup of ginger tea (recipe on page 260) with honey or agave.
- Sit for ten or more minutes in Mindfulness Meditation (page 44).
- Do the winter yin yoga sequence (page 262).
- Brush your skin (page 83), and give yourself a massage with warm sesame oil (page 190), followed by a hot bath. Make this a purification ritual. Say aloud all that you want to wash away.
- For breakfast make the Banana Blueberry Blast Smoothie and the Chia Seed Porridge on page 253, or another hot porridge, along with a cup of ginger tea.
- Prepare the Three-Bean Chili and let it cook for the next two hours.
- Sit for ten minutes, looking out the window practicing the Sky Meditation (page 278).

- Play some of your favorite music. Gather a stack of old magazines and catalogs, and cut out images that reflect the visions that you're incubating this season and wanting to bring to life in the spring. Then glue them onto a sheet of poster board, and hang it above your altar or in your office or bedroom.
- Finish making your lunch — the millet and roasted broccoli (recipes on page 255). Then enjoy your chili, broccoli, and millet while using the conscious eating guidelines from chapter 4.
- Lie down and rest or nap for thirty minutes.
- Choose an inspiring book to read for the next hour. Drink another glass of water.
- Do the hot ginger compress (page 239).
- Sit for ten minutes in Mindfulness Meditation, but instead of focusing on your breath, use sounds as the object of your concentration.
- Do the winter flow yoga practice (page 265).
- Make Kale Chips (recipe on page 258), and enjoy them with some of the leftover millet and chili for dinner.
- Enjoy a cup of ginger tea with honey.
- Spend the evening reading your book or watching an inspirational movie.
- Sit for ten minutes in Mindfulness Meditation.
- 10:00 P.M.: Lights out!

THE HEALING DREAMTIME

Most of us walk around tired all the time. Either our schedules are too full, or we have problems sleeping, or both; but all of us could benefit from more sleep, and winter's the time to do it. Your circadian rhythms shift yet again to mirror those of the earth, and the cold, long nights invite you to slumber deeply in your cave.

Sleep is the most important ingredient for your health and happiness. It's when true healing can happen. Without it your hormones get out of whack — which in turn affects your emotions, your digestion, your metabolism, the way your mind works, your sex drive, your relationships, and even your general outlook. You already know this, though. Don't you always look and feel better after a good night's sleep? That's all the evidence you need. If you're feeling out of sync with your sleep rhythms, use this season to redevelop or strengthen a bedtime ritual (see chapter 2 to review this).

Remember, you need eight to nine hours of sleep at night. Sometimes with family visits and travel around the holidays, this can be difficult to achieve, and you may have to defend the practice viciously! Aside from New Year's Eve, this is not the time of year for late-night parties. If you're sick or run-down, you'll need more like ten hours, maybe even eleven or twelve. This will help you to keep your immunity strong and also to avoid holiday burnout and excess weight gain, because your stress hormones spike when you don't sleep well.

If you do get sick, that's your body's signal that you need to rest. Illness always hands us the opportunity to reevaluate our lives and to do things differently. So when a cold or flu strikes, don't push your way through a workday. Be kind to yourself, and take a "bed day" at home. In fact, even when I'm not sick but just feeling very tired and out of sorts, I take a personal bed day. I stay in bed, sometimes napping, sometimes writing in my journal, reading, looking out the window, working from my laptop, or watching a movie. It reminds me of when I was sick as a little girl and I would camp out in my parents' bed all day, watching game shows and soap operas on TV as my mom brought me hot soup.

WINTER MOON TIME PRACTICES

When you drift off into the dream world each night, especially during the nights of the new moon and your menstruation, take special note of your dreams. Physiologically, dreams signal that you're in a deep sleep, which is the most restorative stage of the rest cycle. Your unconscious mind speaks to you in symbols through your dreams, and learning to understand them can give you valuable messages from your intuitive self for how to implement changes. Plus, your dreams are much more vivid during menstruation. Your spirit is sending you signs for how to bring necessary changes into your life. They're showing you what you need to purify and revamp after menstruation.

Keep a notepad and a pen next to your bed. When you wake up in the middle of the night with a dream, or before you roll out of bed in the morning, jot down as many details as you can remember. You'd be surprised at how accurate your dreams are in reflecting what's happening in your life, as well as signs for how to move forward. A good dream analyst or book can help you learn how to decipher your dreams. Doing so helps to guide you into the watery inner aspects of your being, those that are most hidden, most feminine, most yin — and most vital to your well-being.

TRY THIS

When you honor water, you're honoring the great mother, the Divine Feminine. She is you and you are she, so find ways to conserve and revere her, and teach your family to do the same.

1. Turn off the faucet when you're brushing your teeth. Turn off the shower while you're shaving or lathering in your shampoo.
2. Run the dishwasher and washing machine only when they're completely full.
3. Say no to bottled water. Buy a high-quality water filter and a stainless steel water bottle instead.
4. Honor water as a living entity. Be grateful for it. Place inspiring words or mantras on your glass or water bottle. My water-filled mason jar bears a sticker that says "bliss."
5. Spend time near bodies of water. If you're near a creek or a river, sit on its banks and meditate on its flow. I did this on the banks of the Ganges River, day after day, on my first trip to India.
6. In the bathtub, pool, or hot tub, let yourself just float for three to fifteen minutes. Feel supported. Let go.
7. Limit the number of baths you take to one or two a week, taking showers instead.
8. Swim in saline swimming pools instead of chlorine-laden ones.
9. Use green household cleaners and detergents. Never put chemicals or pharmaceutical drugs down the drain or toilet!
10. Drink a minimum of sixty-four ounces of water a day (more if you're at a high altitude, sick, or detoxing). Keep a glass of water, a cup of herbal tea, or a water bottle with you at all times to help with this. When you get thirsty, your body starts to secrete stress hormones into your bloodstream, and your whole inner equilibrium goes out of whack.
11. Take time-outs during the day to stand up and move your hips. I just got myself a hula hoop to bring fluidity to my hips in the middle of the workday.
12. Appreciate how rejuvenating water can be. Wash away worries in the shower. Baptize yourself again and again in swimming holes, waterfalls, the ocean, and streams.

THE WATER ELEMENT

Water, the dominant element of the winter season, holds the key to your femininity. It's fluid, maternal, versatile, soft, and strong. It, like you, is the source of all life. In utero, we float in a sea of amniotic fluid. Water makes up 70 to 80 percent of our bodies, and the earth herself holds the same percentage, with the chemical composition of her oceans' waters being almost identical to that of human blood plasma.

When the water element lives in balance in your body, you feel connected to the deepest essence of your being, your highest potential. You remember to canoe downstream and follow the current, for when you do so, everything flows. You're going along for the ride, rather than doing the steering. You're adapting and shape-shifting, just as water molds itself into whatever container your pour it into. Flowing like this preserves your energy and reminds you of the power in the mantra "less is more."

I really had to embody the lessons of water in the early months of writing this book, when life took me for a wild ride and I had to completely take my hands off the steering wheel. Within a sixty-day period my boyfriend announced he was moving out of our house (and proceeded to do so), my landlord then told me I needed to move out of my house so he could give it to different tenants, I signed the contract to write this book, and I had a short window to find a new home and complete this manuscript, all the while feeling the intensity of my broken heart. To say I felt overwhelmed and stressed out would be an understatement. I could feel myself spiraling down into my usual method of coping with uncertainty — control. I scoured Craigslist for the right apartment multiple times a day, emailed everyone I knew, went to open houses. I made a list of everything I wanted and needed in a living space and visualized it daily. Nothing. Yet I realized I had a choice. Underneath my frantic attempts, a wise voice deep down was trying to tell me, "Let go. Trust me. Stop the search. I will show you the way."

Eventually I surrendered, and out of the blue one of my best friends called me. She asked me how I was, and I filled her in on the latest events. She couldn't believe the serendipity: she had just bought a new house and was moving out of her current home — a quiet, peaceful refuge in Ashland, Oregon. I could come anytime and stay as long as I needed to. Although I had never been to Ashland, it felt right. I packed my car and drove out there just a few weeks later. I ended up spending six weeks there, getting the space I needed to regroup emotionally and write the first draft of this book before returning to Boulder.

This is the action of water. Obstacles become part of the path that we mold ourselves to and yield around—think of a river flowing over and around rocks, sometimes violently, sometimes sweetly. They don't stop us, and we don't try to remove them or control them. We let them soften us, and we incorporate them into our Way.

Water also governs our emotions. Are they flowing or stagnant? Practice listening to and checking in with yourself as often as you can by asking, "How am I feeling now?" and "Where do I feel this emotion in my body?" and by dropping any story you may have about your emotions and *focusing solely on the sensations that the feeling creates in your body*. On another level, water relates to wisdom and knowledge. It's what calls us to quench our curiosity and desire to live as our best selves through seeking coaches and mentors. In our bodies, water relates to the lymphatic flow, urine, saliva, sweat, tears, and sexual fluids. In the wintertime you can stimulate these by jumping on the trampoline (the lymph system is the only one in the body that doesn't have it's own "pump," so this does the job), taking steam baths and saunas, engaging in vigorous exercise (hot yoga is great this time of year), allowing yourself to cry and make noises as you need to release emotions from your body, and taking time to enjoy intimacy with your partner and yourself. If you're not feeling your sexual mojo, you may be depleted and exhausted. To get these juices flowing again you'll need to get your Zs and offer some support to your kidneys and adrenals.

THE SOURCE OF YOUR SPARKLE

Physiologically, the kidneys and bladder govern the water element and are the dominant organ pair this season. Your kidneys, shaped like ears and residing in your back body, just below and behind your lowest floating rib, filter your blood and keep it clean — imperative for maintaining homeostasis in your body. Your bladder, a muscular organ in your pelvis, receives, stores, and then eliminates urine, one of the by-products of purified blood from the kidneys.

The Chinese considered the bladder to be the storehouse of emotions and the kidneys to hold your vitality and longevity. In fact, your overall sparkle reflects your kidney health. Look at yourself in the mirror today — really look. Is there a dullness there, an unexplored sadness? Or is there vibrancy and a deep connection with your inner self? Also note the color and tone of your skin and the luster of your hair, for these too point to how your kidneys are faring.

If you're facing a chronic illness, an important place to look (and treat) is the energetic state of your kidneys, which a trained traditional Chinese doctor can do through a pulse and tongue diagnosis. Lower-back pain, as well as problems with your reproductive system, such as infertility or impairment to sexual organs or their functions, can also be traced back to your kidney health.

RECOVERING FROM ADRENAL EXHAUSTION

An alarming number of us are walking around with exhausted adrenals. The results of this can be extreme fatigue, accelerated aging, mental fuzziness, weight gain, insomnia, and thyroid disorders. Your adrenals balance more than fifty hormones in your body; support the functioning of your nervous system; reduce inflammation; and balance blood pressure, heartbeat, and sex hormones. If you're always on the run or depending on caffeine or sugar to bolster flagging energy, if you have difficulty getting out of bed in the morning, crave sweet or salty foods, or find yourself weary and irritable, you may need to rebuild your adrenal reserves. Here's how:

- Get at least eight to nine hours of undisturbed sleep each night.
- Take more vitamin C and B (your body burns through these really quickly whenever you're under stress).
- Take herbal blends with astragalus, Cordyceps, eleuthero, rhodiola, and licorice root.
- Find ways to reduce your stress.
- Exercise in the morning.
- Get acupuncture.
- Do more yin yoga (especially the kidney sequence on page 262).
- Get massages.
- Honor daily, weekly, monthly, and yearly cycles of rest and activity.
- Eat more kidney-nourishing foods (more details in the next chapter).
- Cut out or reduce your intake of caffeine, alcohol, and white sugar.

While your kidneys thrive in the extreme cold, these low temperatures can weaken them if you don't keep yourself warm and dry. When you go outside, bundle up appropriately and, as my grandmother (and maybe yours too) told you — don't go outside in the cold with wet hair! In Japan it's common to find "kidney warmers" — these are like giant leg warmers that you wear around your torso to give extra protection to your kidneys.

Strengthening kidney energy requires the key actions of this season: receptivity, deep relaxation, and reflection. Being receptive means being able to listen well to others (the kidneys are also associated with the ear and hearing), as well as being able to listen to your own emotions and to self-soothe, or mother, yourself. When you get out of balance, fear can dominate your emotional landscape. This may show up as phobias, negative thinking or gossip, and even an inability to commit, for strong kidney energy translates as willpower and ambition, unhindered by hesitation. When facing fearful thought patterns it's important to ask yourself, "What inspires me?," "What do I love?," "What do I stand for?," "What legacy do I want to leave?" and then to take a step back and dream up a new world for yourself, guided by your heart.

There are many delicious ways to nurture your kidneys through foods as well, so let's do that now in the kitchen.

REMEMBER

- Spend more time alone this season to rest and reflect. Nurture your dreams.
- Move through your fear of facing your inner darkness. Go inside to find your light. Connect with your heart and womb wisdom.
- Contemplate your relationship to water and to your emotions, and think about whether you tend to go with the flow or try to control life.
- Conserve resources — your energy, electricity, fuel, water, and money.
- Keep warm outside to nurture your kidney energy. Assess your sparkle, and see if you need to boost your inner reservoirs of vitality.

Chapter 19

IN *the* KITCHEN
Staying Warm

 ne of the most crucial ways to nurture and restore your-
self this winter is with your food. This season abounds with family traditions of all sorts, and tasty treats rest at the center of most of these. However, if you're hobnobbing at holiday parties, paring down your exercise regime because it's too cold to go for a run, or feeling generally blue, you may find yourself reaching for not-so-nourishing foods this season. Have faith that there are delicious alternatives to both delight and heal you!

SAD: THE ANNUAL PMS

We've explored how PMS can be brought on by stress. We also experience a more global type of PMS annually through seasonal affective disorder (SAD), a winter depression that sets in, mostly for women, as this cold, dark season descends to show us what isn't working in our lives.

Molly felt this when she moved from California to Michigan when her husband got a new job. Cold and isolated during her first winter there, she didn't yet have a support group to help cheer her up, and she spent a lot of time at home with their toddler.

During our first Skype meeting, I suggested that she have her vitamin D levels checked. Vitamin D (also known as the sunshine vitamin, since sun exposure triggers its production in the body) works a lot as a hormone does in your body. It increases your resistance not only to viruses but also to cancer; and most of us — 53 percent of women, 41 percent of men, and 61 percent of children — have insufficient levels, especially in the dreary wintertime.[1] Low levels of vitamin D have been linked to heart disease, diabetes, chronic pain, and depression. In fact, most cases of SAD can be curbed by bringing your vitamin D levels back up, which you can do by taking a supplement and by getting more sunshine. We all require ten to fifteen minutes of sun exposure at least twice a week on our legs, arms, hands, or back without sunscreen to generate adequate amounts of vitamin D — crucial for the absorption and metabolism of calcium and phosphorus, maintaining a healthy body weight, and regulating the immune system.

I also worked with Molly to make sure she was getting some daily movement (one of the best ways to boost your mood), meeting one new friend a week, having fun by going on a weekly date night with her husband (and even watching a funny movie or TV show when she was alone), and doing "laughter yoga" daily (more about this in the next chapter).

HOW TO SURVIVE TRADITIONAL HOLIDAY FARE

Since outdoor playtime is limited this season (at least for those of us in snowy, foggy, or rainy environments), winter's the perfect time to get creative in the kitchen. Plus, everyone, everywhere, can partake in innovative food preparation to bring a lively, healthy twist to the next holiday gathering — whether it is for the winter solstice; New Year's Eve; Valentine's Day; the Chinese, Vietnamese, or Tibetan New Year; or anything in between.

In winter you need to bring more building foods such as fats and proteins into your repertoire, as well as those ingredients that produce more heat, to help keep you warm. If you eat animal products, this is the season to eat them more (but make sure they're organic). Things like casseroles and soups are also excellent. You can accent these with sprouts or sprouted bread to enliven meals. Favoring blue and black foods such as seaweeds, black beans, chia seeds, blueberries, black sesame seeds, and wild rice helps to strengthen kidney chi too. And, while it's natural to gain some weight this season (don't worry, you'll shed it again in the spring and summer) because the days are simply shorter and there's less active time to burn calories, you want to avoid excess weight gain by not eating too much. Stick to three solid meals a day, and avoid the holiday grazing that's so easy to do when leftovers are hanging around or you're feeling down.

Most of the time hunger signals are actually signs of thirst, so be sure to stay hydrated. Sip hot tea between meals, for instance. Keep listening to what your body wants. Ask, "What am I really hungry for right now?" Maybe it's not food. Perhaps it's to spend some time alone writing in your journal and tinkering with your watercolors if you've had enough family time. Or maybe you really want to get out of the house and chat in a coffeehouse over a hot cup of chai with a girlfriend. Or to bundle up and take a solitary walk in the woods or around the block to get some fresh air.

If you're eating out and socializing, practice self-care by ordering grilled and steamed dishes instead of fried ones. At restaurants I usually get grilled fish and a double side order of veggies, topped with lemon and olive oil. Keep alcohol consumption to a minimum, and instead sip on a single glass of red wine (for women four to six ounces is the medicinal dose) or sparkling water with lemon. Savor and taste the flavors, and chew your food well. Also, be sure not to deny yourself your holiday favorites. When you're biting into that apple pie topped with vanilla ice cream, really be there for the experience. Taste it fully. Delight in it.

WINTER SHOPPING LIST

During the cold weather, stock your pantry with healthy fats such as nuts, seeds, coconut oil, and coconut milk. A good way to get more of these into your diet is to try a tablespoon of coconut oil in your tea or coffee every day. Since coconut is a powerful antimicrobial, it can help keep your immunity strong while also assisting in curbing SAD. Eat lots of dark, leafy greens such as kale and chard too, since these are packed with the medicine of sunlight.

adzuki beans	cranberries
almonds	dark chocolate
apples	dates
black beans	garlic
black pepper	ginger
bok choy	ginseng
broccoli	greens, sturdy (kale and chard)
brown rice	kidney beans
brown rice or quinoa noodles	kimchi (Korean fermented vegetables, without added salt)
buckwheat	
cashews	lentils
cayenne pepper	licorice
celery	millet
chamomile	miso
chestnuts	mung beans

nettles
oats, steel cut or rolled
oranges
pears
pecans
persimmons
pineapple
pomegranates
pumpkins
raisins

roots (beets, sweet potatoes,
   carrots, onions, turnips,
   rutabagas, parsnips)
ruby red grapefruits
sea vegetables (hijiki, kombu,
   dulse, kelp)
sprouts and sprouted breads
walnuts
winter squash

BREAKFAST MENU

* Banana Blueberry Blast Smoothie
* Chia Seed Porridge

BANANA BLUEBERRY BLAST SMOOTHIE

Serves 2

Give yourself a blast of antioxidants from summer's blueberries on a winter morning. The cashews make this really filling and creamy, while the warming spices give it a little bit of a kick and counter the cold fruits. In the really cold areas of the world, this might be too cooling, and it would be better to have a porridge. You be the judge!

1 cup organic frozen blueberries
1 banana, fresh or frozen
1 ¼-inch piece fresh ginger, peeled
2 cups water
1 handful raw cashews
¼ teaspoon vanilla extract
a pinch each of cardamom, cinnamon, and nutmeg
3 to 5 kale leaves
optional: superfoods (see page 95)

Put everything except the kale in the blender and blend well. Make sure to add enough water so all the ingredients are covered. Add the kale and any super-foods that you like. Blend until smooth.

CHIA SEED PORRIDGE

Serves 2

My roommate and I used to have a chia pet in our boarding school dorm room; little did I know that later on the seeds from this whimsical plant would be one of my favorite foods! Chia seeds are loaded with insoluble fiber and healthy fats — making them wonderful immune boosters and happiness makers (healthy fats help serotonin in the brain). Plus, being black, they're nutritive for your kidney chi, and they have the wonderful ability to take on the flavors of whatever you combine them with.

1 cup almond milk (recipe on page 150)
2 tablespoons maple syrup
1 tablespoon coconut oil, melted
pinch of sea salt
pinch of spices such as cinnamon and cardamom
½ cup goji berries, cranberries, or raisins
½ cup chia seeds

In a medium bowl, combine the milk, maple syrup, coconut oil, salt, and spices. Stir. Add the berries or raisins and chia seeds. Stir well and let the mixture sit for 20 minutes or until it has the consistency of pudding. Transfer the porridge to a saucepan and warm it over low heat. To keep the porridge raw, do not heat it above 115°F. To ensure this, test the temperature with your finger, and remove the pan from heat when the porridge becomes uncomfortably hot to the touch.

OTHER BREAKFAST IDEAS

- French toast made with eggs, nondairy milk, and sprouted Ezekiel bread and served with maple syrup.
- Steel-cut or rolled oats with raisins, black sesame seeds, toasted coconut flakes, and raw honey.
- Poached eggs with steamed greens

LUNCH MENU

- Three-Bean Chili
- Millet
- Oven-Roasted Broccoli

THREE-BEAN CHILI

Serves 8 to 10

Strengthening to the kidneys and adrenal glands, beans are usually shaped like kidneys. Coincidence? Their protein promotes growth and grounding, and they're low in fat and good sources of calcium, potassium, iron, zinc, and B vitamins. You can make a big batch of this chili and freeze some for later. Try serving it with some whole-grain sprouted bread.

2 tablespoons olive oil
1 yellow onion, diced
1 clove garlic, minced
1 cup chopped carrot
1 cup chopped celery
1 green bell pepper, seeded and diced
1 tablespoon chili powder
1 teaspoon dried oregano
1 teaspoon dried cumin
1 teaspoon sea salt
black pepper to taste
2 tablespoons tomato paste
½ cup navy beans (soaked overnight)
½ cup adzuki beans (soaked overnight)
½ cup kidney beans (soaked overnight)
6 cups water
1 cup vegetable broth
2 16-ounce cans diced tomatoes
2 tablespoons tamari
¼ cup chopped cilantro or Italian parsley

In a large skillet, heat olive oil. Add onion, garlic, carrot, celery, and bell pepper, and sauté about 5 minutes. Add spices, salt, and pepper, and cook for another few minutes. Add the tomato paste, and stir over heat for 1 minute. Transfer the sautéed mixture to a large pot, then add the beans, water, vegetable broth, and tomatoes. Stir and bring to a boil. Cover and simmer for 2 hours. Stir in tamari. Sprinkle with parsley or cilantro, and serve.

MILLET

Serves 4

Originating in Africa (and a staple of the North African diet), millet is very high in iron. It's also rich in phosphorus and B vitamins. Not only is this versatile grain easy to digest, but it's also quick and easy to prepare. Eat leftovers as a breakfast porridge!

½ cup millet
1½ cups water

Wash millet in a strainer. In a saucepan, combine millet and water and bring to a boil. Do not stir. Lower heat and simmer, covered, for about 25 minutes, until all the water is absorbed. Remove from heat and let sit for about 5 minutes, covered. Fluff with a fork and serve.

OVEN-ROASTED BROCCOLI

Serves 4

One of my favorite side dishes, this brings a little twist to a simple food and is a great complement to almost any meal.

1 bunch broccoli
2 tablespoons olive oil
1 tablespoon tamari or 1 teaspoon sea salt

Preheat the oven to 400°F. Wash and cut the broccoli into florets. In a bowl, toss the broccoli with the olive oil and tamari. Spread on a baking sheet, and roast for about 15 minutes, until tender and lightly browned.

OTHER LUNCH IDEAS

- A bowl of Oven-Roasted Broccoli, millet, hijiki seaweed (soaked), and boiled adzuki beans, drizzled with olive oil and sea salt.
- Lentil soup with Kale Chips (recipe on page 258) and quinoa.
- Roasted sweet potatoes, beets, chickpeas, and parsnips (tossed in olive oil, cumin, and tamari and cooked for 30 to 45 minutes at 400°F). Dip in walnut miso sauce (1 cup walnuts, some water, 1 tablespoon miso blended together).

DINNER MENU

- Miso Soup
- Short-Grain Brown Rice

MISO SOUP

Serves 6

This soup makes a warm, nourishing dish for cold winter nights. It's also chock-full of anticarcinogens, effective in reducing the effects of environmental toxins and providing a powerful immune boost.

1 handful wakame (a thin, stringy seaweed that you can buy dried in the Asian section of your grocery store)
6 cups cold water, divided
1 three-inch piece dried kombu
1 tablespoon sesame oil
1 onion, sliced into thin crescents
1 carrot, cut into matchstick-size pieces
7 tablespoons barley miso or brown rice miso
8 ounces extra-firm tofu, cut into ½-inch cubes
1 bunch kale or collards, sliced thinly
Sliced scallions for garnish

Soak the wakame in 2 cups cold water until soft, about 15 minutes. In a medium pot, combine the kombu with 4 cups water, bring to a simmer, and gently cook for 2 minutes. Add the wakame and the soaking water to the kombu mixture, and leave it on a low simmer. Add sesame oil to a wok or frying pan, and sauté onions and carrots for about 5 minutes, then transfer them to the pot. Bring the soup back to a simmer if necessary, cover, and cook until vegetables are tender, approximately 25 minutes. Place ½ cup liquid from the pot in a small bowl, add the miso, and stir to dissolve. Return this liquid to the pot. Add the tofu and kale or collards, and simmer for a couple minutes. Do not allow soup to boil (this destroys the miso's medicinal microorganisms). Garnish with scallions.

SHORT-GRAIN BROWN RICE

Serves 6

Simple and warming, this brown rice is very fortifying for the body and loaded with B vitamins and magnesium, which help with relaxation. Have leftovers for lunch, or make them into a breakfast porridge.

> 1 cup uncooked short-grain brown rice
> 2½ cups water
> pinch of sea salt
> gomasio to taste

Rinse the rice. Add rice, water, and salt to a pot and cover. Bring to a boil, then reduce heat and simmer for about 1 hour or until all the water is absorbed. Let stand for about 5 minutes and then fluff with a fork. Serve in small bowls, sprinkled with gomasio.

OTHER DINNER IDEAS

- Lasagna made with rice noodles, marinara sauce, spinach, and cashew cream (equal parts cashews and water blended).
- Short-grain brown rice with Oven-Roasted Broccoli and a "red sauce" (soaked sun-dried tomatoes blended with some onion, garlic, veggie stock, and cumin).
- Leftover miso soup with more veggies, such as sweet potato, broccoli, chard, and kale, added in.

SNACK MENU

- Hot Chocolate
- Kale Chips

HOT CHOCOLATE

Serves 2

The quintessential winter comfort treat — for kids and adults alike. Dark chocolate's an important part of any happy woman's life.

2 cups unsweetened almond, rice, or hemp milk
1 tablespoon agave nectar
2 tablespoons unsweetened cocoa powder
1 to 2 pinches nutmeg
¼ teaspoon cinnamon
optional: pinch of cayenne pepper

In a large saucepan, warm the milk over medium heat. Add agave and stir until dissolved. Add cocoa and whisk until blended. Heat until slightly thick, about 5 minutes. Whisk in spices. Enjoy!

DARK CHOCOLATE

The food that loves to love you back, dark chocolate's loaded with magnesium, manganese, copper, zinc, phosphorus, and antioxidants. These help to keep your heart healthy and your bones strong, and they even help to hydrate your skin, lower your blood pressure, and keep your thinking sharp. Plus, it's a sensual pleasure: eating a piece (about a quarter ounce) a day (make sure it's at least 70 percent cocoa), can be the perfect afternoon pick-me-up that delivers with it a boost of ecstatic delight. I have a little bit almost every day!

KALE CHIPS

Serves 4

These give you the crisp, salty fix that you crave when you reach for the pretzels or potato chips. But instead of fat and sodium, they're packed with iron, calcium, and fiber.

1 large bunch curly green kale
2 tablespoons fresh lemon juice
1 tablespoon nutritional yeast
1 tablespoon tahini
1 teaspoon onion powder
1 tablespoon tamari

Preheat the oven to 350°F. Tear kale stems away (and compost them), then tear leaves into large pieces and put them into a large bowl. In a small bowl, mix together the lemon juice, nutritional yeast, tahini, onion powder, and tamari.

Pour this mixture onto the kale. Using your hands, massage the mixture into the kale leaves, squeezing and tossing the leaves as you go, to help soften them. Mix until leaves are evenly coated. Spread the kale out as flat as possible onto a couple of baking sheets lined with parchment paper. Bake for 15 to 20 minutes, or until kale becomes crisp. Keep a close eye on the kale at the end of its cooking process to make sure it doesn't burn.

TIP: To make this a raw snack, if you have a dehydrator, warm it to 115°F. Spread the kale out onto 4 dehydrator sheets, and dehydrate for 10 to 12 hours or until crisp.

DESSERT MENU

- Gingerbread

GINGERBREAD

Serves 6

A traditional holiday treat that's so healthy you can even eat it for breakfast!

2 cups gluten-free flour mix
½ teaspoon baking soda
2 teaspoons dried ginger
1 teaspoon cinnamon
1 teaspoon nutmeg
1 teaspoon ground cloves
1 teaspoon ground black pepper
½ cup agave nectar
⅔ cup unsweetened almond, rice, or hemp milk
¼ cup molasses
1 egg (or place 1 tablespoon chia seeds in a cup, and add 3 tablespoons water. Allow the mixture to sit for about 15 minutes. ¼ cup hydrated chia seeds equals approximately 1 egg.)
½ cup coconut oil, plus more for oiling pan

Preheat oven to 350°F. Combine dry ingredients in a bowl, and mix together well with a wooden spoon. Combine wet ingredients in a bowl, and do the same.

Gradually add the wet to the dry, blending with a mixer on medium speed until the batter is smooth. Grease a loaf pan with the extra coconut oil, and pour in batter. Bake for about an hour, until risen and firm.

THE GOODNESS OF GINGER ROOT

I enjoy ginger year-round, but I enjoy it the most during the winter. For centuries, it's been the go-to root for boosting immunity, for easing nausea related to motion and morning sickness, and for treating GI disturbances (such as constipation, gas, and indigestion). You can sip some ginger tea throughout the day to help you keep warm. Having a little bit before, during, and after meals will help your digestion. When you have a cold, add honey and fresh lemon for a soothing treat. It's also great for suppressed menstruation.

To make ginger tea, chop 3 to 4 inches of a root into fine pieces (or pound in a large mortar). Put in a large pot of water. Bring to a boil, and then simmer for 15 to 30 minutes.

Now let's look at ways you can stay active this season through yoga while also honing your courage and your capacity to look inward and grow your feminine intuition.

REMEMBER

- You'll gravitate toward more proteins, fats, and carbohydrates during the winter. These help to keep you warm, and it's natural to put on some weight this season.
- Keep listening to your body. Ask, "What am I really hungry for?"
- Eat slowly and mindfully so you can tell when you're truly satisfied.
- Supplement your diet with vitamin D, and get outside into the sun whenever you can.
- Sip on hot ginger tea to keep you warm and well.
- Share your healthy treats with friends and family at holiday gatherings — or even host your own.

Chapter 20

ON *the* YOGA MAT

Deep Rest

It's so easy to fall into a winter funk, and movement's the best way to shake it, regardless of the season. So although it's not bathing-suit season (unless you live in a warm climate or go on a tropical vacation), and though it's a good thing to allow your energy levels to be lower, you still need to get moving every day. Do both: fall into quieter practices by doing more forward bends, and also shake things up. If you have a mini-trampoline, now's the time to dust it off. Set it up in your office, and take a five-minute jumping break to your favorite music (I know it's cheesy, but I love to do it to the Pointer Sisters' "Jump"). This gets your lymph moving, and you'll feel much lighter and more enthusiastic afterward.

Be sure to balance this activity with lots of self-care: get plenty of sleep, give and receive hugs (I've heard that we need twelve hugs a day to be happy), get massages, and take hot baths, saunas, and steams. Remember, winter's the wisdom season. Use the surrounding darkness as inspiration to go within and find the light there. Trust that which you cannot see but know in your heart to be true. Listen to your body. When a friend asks you to go to a movie and dinner, do you feel excitement or an inner pulling away? Would you rather spend a quiet evening at home but are afraid to hurt her feelings? Your body never lies. Use the stillness around you to delve into your inner world. Believe in your dreams. Listen to the whispers in your heart.

This season's yoga and meditation practices will help you to balance dynamic movement with restorative stillness. The winter, the final spoke of the year, invites you to blend your inner and outer worlds to give rise to knowledge, wisdom, and clear guidance that are your birthright as a woman. The cultivation of these qualities allows you to come full circle, to harness the lessons you've learned over the year and let them percolate deep inside so they're ready to ripen into action and a more evolved version of you in the spring.

Since energy can be at a real low this season and schedules can get chaotic with holiday travel and gatherings, keep in mind that any time's a good time to practice! If you have a full hour, great. If not, don't let that stop you. Even a five-minute break with some Cat/Cow movements of the spine and Downward-Facing Dog can completely shift your energy. Don't underestimate the power of doing less. Also, as you did in the fall, try to raise your body temperature when you do the flow practice so that you break a sweat. Turn the heat up, wear layers, or practice next to a space heater or fireplace. You need to keep the flame burning so that water keeps flowing and doesn't become stagnant in your body — the signs of which are melancholy, laziness, bloating, delayed or scanty menstruation, uterine or ovarian cysts and fibroids, and stiff, achy muscles and joints.

EMOTIONAL AND MENTAL QUALITIES OF THE KIDNEYS AND BLADDER

The kidney-bladder duo orchestrates the balance between yin and yang energy throughout the whole body, especially governing all things related to birth and change. They house the reserves of your vitality, so treating this pair will help to address any imbalance or disturbance in your body.

Fear arises when the kidneys are out of balance, and, likewise, when we feel fear or anxiety we are placing an extra burden on them. Mentally, you may find yourself having a hard time following through on projects through a lack of personal power and enthusiasm. However, when kidney chi is harmonious, you will feel grounded, soft, and connected to your innate wisdom. You'll have the energy and motivation to complete what you've started, and you'll feel more energetic, sensual, and sexual.

WINTER YIN YOGA

With winter being the most yin part of the yearly cycle, you might find it easier to get still and quiet now than at other times of the year. This yin practice plays a crucial role in strengthening your kidney energy and therefore in replenishing your life force. One of the wonderful things about yin yoga is that it doesn't require much energy to do. That makes it perfect for when you're sick, exhausted, or menstruating. It provides healing energy without depleting your scarce reserves.

The poses that follow gently stimulate your kidney and bladder meridians. The former starts in the baby toe of each foot, travels through the arches and

YOGA NIDRA

On days when you're feeling really run-down, take thirty minutes (it's great to do after lunch) for Yoga Nidra. More than thirty years ago, Swami Satyananda Saraswati, founder of the renowned Bihar School of Yoga in eastern India, adapted ancient tantric meditation techniques into a practice he called Yoga Nidra, which translates as "psychic sleep." This practice induces complete relaxation while you maintain consciousness. Here, our deepest levels of creativity and healing energies can awaken. In this state one can ultimately change thought patterns — and even the personality — for the better. This practice has been shown even to alleviate PTSD in war veterans. But even if healing deep trauma's not your aim, you will be happy to know that you will emerge from Yoga Nidra feeling rested and ready to engage with the world. (A twenty- to thirty-minute session of Yoga Nidra is said to be the equivalent of approximately three hours of deep sleep!).

up the inner legs, and enters the torso through the tailbone, where it runs up along either side of the spine. From there, different branches then flow through the kidneys and bladder as well as the belly, chest, liver, diaphragm, and lungs, ending at the back of the tongue. The latter starts at the outer corners of the eyes, arcs over the head, goes through the brain, and then runs down either side of the spine. One branch moves internally to the kidneys and bladder, and another flows down the backs of the legs to end at the outside of the baby toes.

As you do these practices (or any time you're relaxing), you can massage the origin of the kidney meridian on the sole of your foot. Just to the inside, lower portion of the ball of your foot, you can palpate "Kidney 1," or the "Bubbling Spring" — the only acupuncture point on the bottom of the foot. When you feel around the whole arc alongside the ball, you will most likely come across a very sensitive point. That's Kidney 1. Using your thumb (or a knuckle for more pressure), press into this point for a few seconds to stimulate the kidney meridian.

Before Beginning: Review the sections "Create a Sacred Space" (page 67) and "Yin Yoga" (page 49).

Intention: To deeply rest and restore. To grow quiet so that you can listen to your innermost wisdom.

Total Practice Time: 60 minutes

Full Sequence of Illustrations: Page 264

WINTER YIN YOGA SEQUENCE

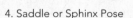

1. Check-In and Intention
2. Belly Breathing
3. Butterfly Pose
4. Saddle or Sphinx Pose

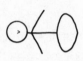
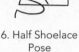

5. Dragonfly Pose
6. Half Shoelace Pose
7. Full Forward Fold
8. Happy Baby Pose

9. Supine Butterfly Pose
10. Equanimity Meditation
11. Dedication of Merit

1. *Check-In and Intention* (2 to 3 minutes): You can review these in chapter 3.
2. *Belly Breathing* (2 to 5 minutes): Place your hands on your belly, just below your belly button. Drop your breath down into your belly, and take some deep breaths in and out. Feel a heaviness in your pelvis, like the darkness of winter. At the same time, connect with the levity in your chest, like the brilliance of summer. Continue taking some deep belly breaths, feeling your body hold these two opposing energies simultaneously. Use this same belly breathing throughout the practice to encourage deep relaxation.
3. *Butterfly Pose* (5 minutes): See page 164.
4. *Saddle* or *Sphinx Pose* (5 minutes): See page 212. *Note:* If you have any lower-back or knee pain, please play it safe and practice Sphinx Pose instead of Saddle.
5. *Dragonfly Pose* (5 minutes): See page 112.
6. *Half Shoelace Pose* (5 minutes on each side): From Dragonfly Pose, bring your legs together. Fold your left knee over your right, keeping your right leg straight. Stay upright, or fold forward. Repeat on the other side.

7. *Full Forward Fold* (5 minutes): See page 165.
8. *Happy Baby Pose* (5 minutes): See page 126. To come out, draw your knees into your chest for a few breaths in Seed Pose (page 124).
9. *Supine Butterfly Pose* (5 minutes): See page 112.
10. *Equanimity Meditation* (5 to 30 minutes): Cross your legs (the other leg on top now), and follow the meditation instructions at the end of this chapter.
11. *Dedication of Merit* (1 minute): Please review instructions on page 52.

MINI-WINTER YIN PRACTICE

Short on time? String these three poses together for a twenty-minute practice. Try them during your lunch break, as your child naps, before your morning shower, or just before sleep.

1. Butterfly Pose
2. Saddle or Sphinx Pose
3. Dragonfly Pose

WINTER FLOW YOGA

This dynamic practice boosts circulation and your metabolism, nourishes your kidney yang chi, and helps to maintain bodily strength, especially in your core. Emotionally and mentally, it reminds you to flow with the larger river of life, your breath, during easeful and challenging moments alike.

Before Beginning: Review the sections "Create a Sacred Space" (page 67) and "Yang (or Flow) Yoga" (page 50).

Intention: To keep your body and emotions fluid by tending to your inner fire.

Total Practice Time: 60 minutes

Full Sequence of Illustrations: Pages 266–69

1. *Check-In and Intention* (2 to 5 minutes): Please revisit chapter 3 for details.
2. *Seated Forward Stretch* (5 breaths in each position): From a seated cross-legged position, bow forward and stretch your arms along the floor. Keep your sitting bones rooted. Then walk your hands over to your left so that your belly's angled over your left knee. Walk your hands over to your right, and do the same thing. Complete this with five more breaths in the center.

WINTER FLOW YOGA SEQUENCE

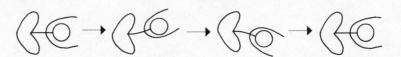

1. Check-In
and Intention

2. Seated Forward Stretch

3. Seated Torso
Circles

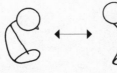

4. Seated Cat   Seated Cow

5. Seated Lateral
Stretch

6. Seated Neck
Stretches

7. Windshield Wipers

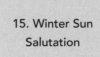

8. Thread the Needle

9. Toe Stretch

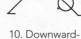

10. Downward-
Facing Dog

11. Standing
Forward Fold

12. Spinal Waves

13. Hip Circles

14. Standing
Lateral Stretch

**15. Winter Sun
Salutation**

Mountain Pose

WINTER FLOW YOGA SEQUENCE *(CONTINUED)*

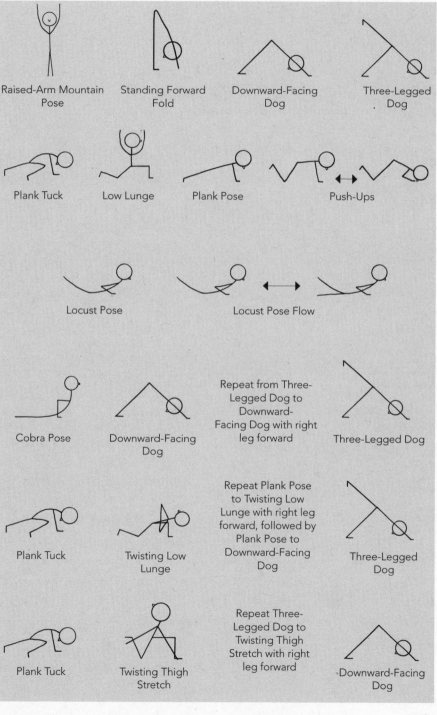

Raised-Arm Mountain Pose

Standing Forward Fold

Downward-Facing Dog

Three-Legged Dog

Plank Tuck

Low Lunge

Plank Pose

Push-Ups

Locust Pose

Locust Pose Flow

Cobra Pose

Downward-Facing Dog

Repeat from Three-Legged Dog to Downward-Facing Dog with right leg forward

Three-Legged Dog

Plank Tuck

Twisting Low Lunge

Repeat Plank Pose to Twisting Low Lunge with right leg forward, followed by Plank Pose to Downward-Facing Dog

Three-Legged Dog

Plank Tuck

Twisting Thigh Stretch

Repeat Three-Legged Dog to Twisting Thigh Stretch with right leg forward

Downward-Facing Dog

WINTER FLOW YOGA SEQUENCE *(CONTINUED)*

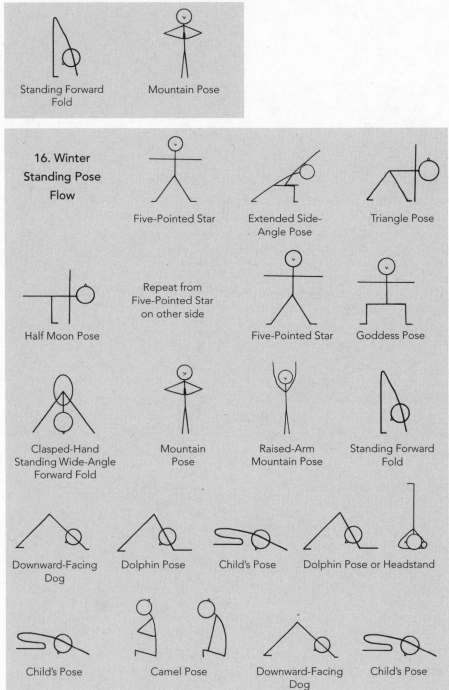

Standing Forward
Fold

Mountain Pose

**16. Winter
Standing Pose
Flow**

Five-Pointed Star

Extended Side-
Angle Pose

Triangle Pose

Half Moon Pose

Repeat from
Five-Pointed Star
on other side

Five-Pointed Star

Goddess Pose

Clasped-Hand
Standing Wide-Angle
Forward Fold

Mountain
Pose

Raised-Arm
Mountain Pose

Standing Forward
Fold

Downward-Facing
Dog

Dolphin Pose

Child's Pose

Dolphin Pose or Headstand

Child's Pose

Camel Pose

Downward-Facing
Dog

Child's Pose

WINTER FLOW YOGA SEQUENCE *(CONTINUED)*

17. Winter Core Flow

Curl-Ups

Hip Lifts

Laughing Bicycle

18. Winter Floor Flow

Constructive Rest Pose

Supine Single-Leg Stretch

Wind-Relieving Pose

One-Knee Spinal Twist

Repeat Single-Leg Stretch to One-Knee Spinal Twist on right side

Seed Pose

19. Final Relaxation Pose

20. Alternate Nostril Breathing

21. Equanimity Meditation

22. Dedication of Merit

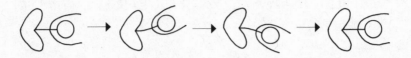

3. *Seated Torso Circles* (5 times in both directions): From an upright seated position, change the cross of your legs. Rest your hands on your thighs, and circle your rib cage to the right, and then to the left.

4. *Seated Cat/Cow* (5 times): From a seated cross-legged position, exhale and round forward, tucking your chin in toward your chest. Inhale, and arch your spine as you look up.

5. *Seated Lateral Stretch* (5 breaths on each side): Sitting upright, put your left hand on the floor beside you. Inhale and stretch your right arm up toward the sky. Exhale and bend over to the left. Inhale up, and on the exhale, repeat to the other side.

6. *Seated Neck Stretches* (5 breaths on each side): Stretch your left arm slightly behind you, out to the side. Keep your hand off the ground, and bend your head over your right shoulder until you feel a stretch along the left side of your neck. Inhale up, and on the exhale, repeat on the other side.

 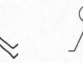

7. *Windshield Wipers* (5 times each side): Uncross your legs, bend your knees, and plant your feet in front of you mat width apart. Place your hands behind you, and lean into them. Inhale, and on the exhale, drop your knees to the left. Inhale and bring them back to center, and on the exhale, drop them over to your right. Then, the next time they're over at the left, inhale and lift your hips off the ground, so you're supported by your left hand and your shins. Stretch your right arm across the right side of your face. Exhale down, and inhale up to the other side.

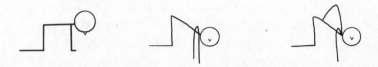

8. *Thread the Needle* (5 breaths on each side): Come onto your hands and knees. Put your weight onto your left hand; as you inhale stretch your right arm up to the sky. Exhale and weave your right arm underneath your left elbow, taking your right ear and shoulder to the ground. *Advanced students:* Inhale, and lift your left arm up, and on the exhale wrap it behind you, taking hold of the top of your right thigh. Repeat on the other side.

9. *Toe Stretch* (5 breaths): From hands and knees, curl your toes under and rest your hips on your heels. Now, inhale up so you're sitting on your heels. *Advanced students:* Interlace your fingers, stretch your arms up, and flip your palms up so they face the ceiling, lifting up through your torso.

10. *Downward-Facing Dog* (5 breaths): See page 118.

11. *Standing Forward Fold* (5 breaths): See page 118.

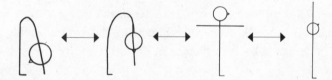

12. *Spinal Waves* (5 times): From Standing Forward Fold, bend your knees softly. Keep your fingertips and the crown of your head heavy. Slowly roll yourself up to standing, letting your spine round and then unfurl. When your spine is upright, take your arms out to the sides and all the way overhead. Let your head be the last thing to come up. Then make your way back down into Standing Forward Fold by lowering your arms, tucking your chin, and letting your vertebrae roll down until your head reaches toward the ground again. Do this a few more times. Come up as you inhale, and go down as you exhale. Finish in a standing position.

13. *Hip Circles* (5 times in each direction): Take your feet as wide as your mat, and place your hands on your hips. Bend your knees slightly, and make wide circles with your hips to the left. Repeat in the other direction.

14. *Standing Lateral Stretch* (5 breaths in each direction): Take your feet hip width apart again. Take your left hand to your left hip. Inhale and lift your right arm up, and exhale over to the left side. Inhale back to center and repeat on the other side.

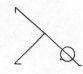

15. *Winter Sun Salutation*
    - *Mountain Pose* (5 breaths): See page 119.
    - *Raised-Arm Mountain Pose* (5 breaths): Inhale into it. See page 171.
    - *Standing Forward Fold* (5 breaths). Exhale into it.
    - *Downward-Facing Dog* (5 breaths): Exhale into it. Step or jump back.
    - *Three-Legged Dog* (5 breaths): Inhale and lift left leg up first. See page 170.
    - *Plank Tuck:* From Three-Legged Dog, exhale, as you take your shoulders forward over your wrists into Plank Pose as you round your back and draw your left knee in toward your chest.

    - *Low Lunge* (5 breaths): Left leg forward. See page 120.
    - *Plank Pose* (5 breaths): See page 120.
    - *Push-Ups* (3)*:* Knees up or down. See page 120.
    - *Locust Pose* (5 breaths): Facedown on the ground, slide the heels of your hands back so they're in line with the base of your rib cage.

    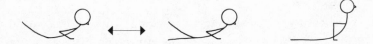

    Inhale, and lift your chest and your legs. Keep the back of your neck long, legs hip width apart, toes spread.
    - *Locust Pose Flow* (5 times): Stay in Locust Pose. As you inhale, stretch your legs wide apart, keeping them straight and your toes spread. As you exhale, draw your legs together.
    - *Cobra Pose* (5 breaths): Keep your chest up, and on the exhale, lower your legs down, hip width apart.
    - *Downward-Facing Dog* (5 breaths).
    - *Three-Legged Dog* (5 breaths): Inhale into it. Right leg up.
    - Repeat the above instructions from Plank Tuck with the right leg forward to Downward-Facing Dog.

- *Three-Legged Dog* (5 breaths): Left leg up.
- *Plank Tuck:* Exhale.
- *Twisting Low Lunge* (5 breaths): Left leg forward. Come into High Lunge Twist (see page 121) with the back knee down.

- Repeat Plank Pose to Twisting Low Lunge with the right leg forward, followed by Plank Pose through Downward-Facing Dog.
- *Three-Legged Dog* (5 breaths): Left leg up.
- *Plank Tuck.*
- *Twisting Thigh Stretch* (5 breaths): Left leg forward. From low lunge, take your right hand to the ground on the inside of your left foot. Inhale and lift your left arm up, and as you exhale, reach it back behind you and twist to look over your left shoulder. *Advanced students:* Bend your right leg, reach back, and take hold of your right foot with your left hand.

- Repeat Three-Legged Dog through Twisting Thigh Stretch with the right leg forward.
- *Downward Facing Dog* (5 breaths).
- *Standing Forward Fold* (5 breaths).
- *Mountain Pose* (5 breaths).

16. *Winter Standing Pose Flow*
    - *Five-Pointed Star* (5 breaths): See page 173.
    - *Extended Side-Angle Pose* (5 breaths): Left side first. See page 122.
    - *Triangle Pose* (5 breaths): See page 122.
    - *Half Moon Pose* (5 breaths): See page 173.
    - Repeat from Five-Pointed Star on the other side.
    - *Five-Pointed Star* (5 breaths).
    - *Goddess Pose* (10 breaths): From Five-Pointed Star, exhale and turn your toes out slightly. Bend your knees so that they're in line with your second toes. Take your arms out to your sides. Stretch your arms and fingertips out along the horizon as if they're coming straight from your heart. Lengthen your lower back down toward your heels. Make any noises that you want — growl, groan, howl...
    - *Clasped-Hand Standing Wide-Angle Forward Fold* (5 breaths): From Goddess Pose, turn your feet back in so the outer edges are parallel. Exhale, and interlace your fingers behind your back. Inhale and lift

your chest up; exhale and fold over. To come out, exhale and place your hands on your hips, and on the inhale, come up to stand.

- *Mountain Pose* (5 breaths).
- *Raised-Arm Mountain Pose* (5 breaths).
- *Standing Forward Fold* (5 breaths).
- *Downward-Facing Dog* (5 breaths).
- *Dolphin Pose* (10 breaths): From Downward-Facing Dog, lower your forearms to the ground, and interlace your fingers, palms slightly apart. Keep your elbows right under your shoulders. Move your armpits forward toward your fingers as you move your chest toward your thighs. Keep your head off the ground. *Advanced students:* Walk your feet in closer toward your face, keeping your spine long.
- *Child's Pose* (10 breaths).
- *Dolphin Pose* or *Headstand* (10 to 30 breaths): See instructions for headstand on page 223. *Note:* If you're menstruating, you can rest in Child's Pose or Supine Butterfly Pose (page 112).
- *Child's Pose* (10 breaths).
- *Camel Pose* (5 to 10 breaths; repeat 3 times): Come up to kneeling, with knees hip width apart, toes curled under. Exhale and place your palms on your lower back, fingers pointing down, elbows squeezing in. Inhale and lift your chest. Exhale and lengthen your tailbone down to the ground as you arch backward. *Advanced students:* Take your hands down to your heels.
- *Downward-Facing Dog* (5 breaths).
- *Child's Pose* (5 breaths).

17. *Winter Core Flow*

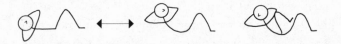

- *Curl-Ups* (20 to 30 times in each direction): Come onto your back, and place your feet on the ground, hip width apart, right under your knees. Hold the back of your head lightly with your hands. Keep your elbows away from your face. Draw your belly button toward your spine, flatten your low back to the ground, and keep it there. Exhale to curl up. Inhale to lower down. Hold the same position as above, but as you exhale, twist each elbow to the opposite knee.

- *Hip Lifts* (10 to 30 times): Stretch your legs up toward the ceiling. Flex your toes toward your knees. Keep your hands facing down next to your hips. As you exhale, lift your hips off the ground so your feet reach straight up. Don't use momentum; try to use your lower abdominal muscles. Inhale and lower your hips back down.

- *Laughing Bicycle* (1 minute): Draw your knees into your chest, and circle your legs in the air as if you're riding a bicycle. Start laughing — even if the laughter's forced. Keep going!

LAUGHTER YOGA

It seems silly, but that's the point! Dr. Madan Kataria, a physician from Mumbai, India, launched the first Laughter Club in 1995, and today there are more than sixty thousand Social Laughter Clubs around the world. The premise is that anyone can laugh for no reason whatsoever and that doing so is crucial in generating feelings of happiness and pleasure. In other words, you can make happiness a daily practice, no matter how you're feeling. One of my favorite tidbits of wisdom is "fake it till you make it." Even if you're feeling blue, give yourself a pick-me-up with some laughter yoga.

18. *Winter Floor Flow*
- *Constructive Rest Pose* (5 breaths): See page 125.
- *Supine Single-Leg Stretch* (5 breaths): From Constructive Rest Pose, draw your left knee in toward your chest. Extend your right leg straight on the ground, toes pointing up toward the ceiling. Interlace your fingers behind your left thigh, and stretch that leg up toward the ceiling. Press your thigh into your hands as you also try to draw that leg toward you. Create space in the front of the left hip and through your left kidney.

- *Wind-Relieving Pose* (5 breaths): Draw your left knee in toward your chest, holding the shin with both hands. As you do this, stretch your right leg straight along the ground.
- *One-Knee Spinal Twist* (5 breaths on each side): See page 112.
- Repeat Single-Leg Stretch to One-Knee Spinal Twist on the right side.
- *Seed Pose* (5 breaths): See page 124.

19. *Final Relaxation Pose* (5 to 10 minutes): See page 126.

20. *Alternate Nostril Breathing* (5 minutes): Come to a comfortable seated posture. Rest with your palms facing up on your thighs. Close your eyes, and enjoy some deep belly breathing. Lift your right arm up, and fold your index and middle finger in toward your palm. Then close off your left nostril with your right ring finger. Inhale through your right nostril. Keep your fingers there, but release their hold on the nostril. Then close your right nostril with your right thumb and exhale through the left. Now inhale through the left and exhale through the right. Alternate right and left for about 5 minutes. Be sure to always inhale through the same nostril from which you just exhaled. Make your inhales and exhales about 5 counts each.

     This breath balances the lunar and solar energies in your body, keeping your body and mind in a state of equanimity. When breath flows freely through both channels, we stay in rhythm with the sun energy of the day and the moon energy of the night.

21. *Equanimity Meditation* (5 to 30 minutes): Read instructions on the next page.

22. *Dedication of Merit* (1 minute): Please review instructions on page 52.

MINI-WINTER FLOW PRACTICE

If you're short on time, you can do this practice in fifteen to twenty minutes:

1. Seated Cat/Cow (5 times)
2. Thread the Needle (5 breaths on each side)
3. Winter Sun Salutation (1 to 3 rounds)
4. Extended Side-Angle Pose (5 breaths each side)
5. Dolphin Pose or Headstand (10 to 30 breaths)
6. Child's Pose (5 breaths)
7. One-Knee Spinal Twist (5 breaths)
8. Seed Pose (5 breaths)
9. Final Relaxation (2 to 3 minutes)

EQUANIMITY MEDITATION

Equanimity might be the hardest of the four heavenly abodes to truly realize, but it's worth practicing because from equanimity true wisdom and happiness can arise. In fact, it's only from equanimity that you can authentically feel and express loving-kindness, joy, and compassion. If you're caught up in rage, revenge, or self-pity, you're at the whim of your emotions and unable to act from your highest self.

While sometimes people confuse equanimity with dullness or apathy, that's actually quite the opposite of what it means. Other words for equanimity include *steadiness, evenness of mind*, and *composure*. Equanimity requires dynamic spaciousness — not getting entangled in the things we want (pleasure, praise, recognition, gain) or in the things we *don't* want (pain, blame, disrepute, loss). It means feeling deeply without getting swept away by emotion or circumstance. In each moment, you can choose to feel and reside in your emotions without acting out or repressing them. You can stamp your feet and raise your voice when you're angry without blaming or judging the person you're with. This trains you to *respond* rather than to *react*, and it takes discernment and skill.

Here are some simple ways to let equanimity emerge: If you're having an argument with someone, go for a walk or do something else that's physical (scream in your car, punch your pillow, dance to music with lots of drums). Once you've released that fire, come back and continue your conversation. If you want to blame or judge someone, take a moment to feel your feet on the ground, and draw in some deep breaths. Ask yourself, "How is this person a reflection of me?," "What lesson is she here to teach me?," "What role have I played in this scenario?"

At the end of a yoga class many years ago, my teacher instructed us to experience the present moment from the part of ourselves that hadn't changed at all since we were small children. As you read these words, sense that place within yourself too. For me it was a part of me that didn't care what kind of day I had had or how I looked or felt. It was something much vaster, much freer. It was awareness itself, and it has been with me during each moment of my life.

From connecting with that open, aware part of myself, whenever I feel like I'm getting pigeonholed into narrow thinking (any form of emotional suffering is a sure sign of this), I remember to take a bird's-eye view, to see the bigger picture, just as an eagle would see the patterns of a city's streets rather than a traffic jam. When we develop the capacity to rest more in our spacious awareness than in our needs, wants, and momentary obsessions, a real heartiness of spirit emerges. We're not as prone to getting knocked down when things don't go our way. The following practice helps you to develop equanimity. I particularly like this one because anyone, anywhere, can do it. It's called the Sky Meditation.

1. Choose a time when the sun is not too bright in the sky. Early morning and evening are best.

2. Sit down outside or near a window. You can also lie down on the grass. If you're sitting down, make sure that you have mostly sky in your line of sight.

3. Relax your gaze, relax your body, and let your jaw drop open slightly, as if you're in a state of quiet awe.

4. Sit for five minutes, letting your awareness mix with the spaciousness of the sky. You're not looking for anything or trying to get anywhere. You're just gazing at the sky.

5. Can the sky remind you of anything about who you truly are, beyond your thoughts and feelings?

6. Blink whenever you need to, and remember to never look directly at the sun.

7. When you've finished, close your eyes, take a few deep breaths, and prepare to transition into the rest of your day, keeping that sense of vast awareness with you during all your thoughts, conversations, and actions.

8. Take a moment to contemplate the benefits you experience from balance and equanimity — in your body, mind, emotions, and actions.

REMEMBER

-   Balance solar and lunar energies this season. Treat your body to some movement every day, and temper that with adequate rest and time for reparation.

-   Remember that five minutes of yoga and/or meditation is better than none at all! If you don't have time to do five Sun Salutations, do one. A little bit goes a long way.

-   Bring some laughter into your life every day: watch a silly movie or TV show, or do some laughter yoga.

-   Gaze out the window at the sky. Watch the clouds moving. Sense the contrast between that which is vast and omnipresent and that which is moving and changing.

Chapter 21

WINTER REFLECTIONS

When I attend silent meditation retreats — or even when I took a step back from my life to write this book — I can cycle through a whole range of feelings, from deep peace and contentment to feeling as if I must be the most neurotic person on the planet. In the same way, when you hold a yin yoga posture, deep emotions can surface and you become more aware of your thoughts. When you slow down, you notice more. You feel more. This is a good thing.

Becoming wise doesn't mean eradicating your idiosyncrasies and imperfections. It means making peace with them, owning them, and wearing them on your sleeve because they're what make you *you*. As your body starts to relax and you drop into more of a spacious place of awareness, you might notice deep beliefs such as "Everyone else does it better than me," "Nobody likes me," or any tune from the "I'm not good enough" soundtrack bubbling up more strongly.

Now's the time to make equanimity your ally. Stand with dignity in the truth of your body's present experience and participate in the moment. Oh, yes, my socks feel warm on my feet, and the tiles are cool beneath me. I hear a crow outside. My belly's rumbling. Despite all the changes you've gone through in the past year, your capacity to abide in the present moment and stay open to it, regardless of what you're thinking and feeling, has increased. Your direct experience has taught you to trust cycles in the depths of your being.

From this place of paying attention to life and opening to it, you can formulate your dreams and desires for the coming year. Not only that, but you are now more open to receive, enjoy, and participate in life's blessings as they get ready to perfume your life this spring and beyond.

COMMUNITY RITUAL

Here are some simple steps to help you practice the art of presence, equanimity, and listening:

1. Invite a friend, relative, or intimate partner to practice compassionate listening with you.
2. Sit down on the floor or on chairs facing each other in a quiet room. You can hold hands, if that feels right.
3. Set a timer for ten minutes and decide who will go first.
4. Look into each other's eyes. The first person speaks for ten minutes without stopping. Begin by speaking about the sensations in your body, and go from there.
5. The partner does not nod, say "uh-huh," or do anything other than look the person who is speaking in the eye, listening deeply.
6. After ten minutes, stay in a space of silence and connect with your breath, and then switch roles.
7. When you've finished, thank each other in any way that feels appropriate.

Now, looking back over the past few months, think about how things have been for you, both in your outer and inner worlds, and explore them in your journal through the questions below:

MONTH ONE

1. At the start of this season, I felt afraid of:
2. My main health concerns were:
3. The three main ways that I habitually react to fear are:
4. I usually cope with the stress of family visits and the holiday season by _____, but right now I'm interested in cultivating a new response of _____ or _____.
5. The one habit I'm going to focus on cultivating for the next thirty days is _____. I will omit _____ in order to create space for this. The main things I hope to experience as a result of this are:

MONTH TWO

1. I have learned to trust the wisdom of my womb and intuition more this season through _____ and _____. This is reflected in my outer life through _____ and _____. The results I'm feeling are mostly _____ and _____.

2. The three words I'd use to describe my connection with my deepest wisdom right now are: _____, _____, and _____. Ideally, those three words would be: _____, _____, and _____.

3. Some ways that I'm finding it helpful to respond rather than react are:

4. What's brought me the greatest sense of ease this month is:

5. On a scale of 1 to 10 (with 1 being cool as a cucumber and 10 being about to explode), my current stress level is _____. Ideally, it would be _____. Some things I can do to help myself to unwind are _____ and _____. Some people I can ask for support from are _____ and _____.

MONTH THREE

1. What I'm celebrating most from my efforts this season are:

2. Looking back, I realize that my biggest challenges were:

3. I experienced some dark nights of the soul when _____ and also when _____. The light and lessons I received from embracing those experiences fully were:

4. When I think back to the times in my life when I was the most vibrant and rested, the following memories come to mind:

5. The vision for myself and my life in this next year that's becoming clear to me now is:

Having now cycled through all the seasons of the year, you have completed your initiation into becoming a wise woman. Because of your courage to face all parts of yourself, you embody a fierce yet gentle presence. Just being who you are serves as a light and inspiration for others. You have found your way home to yourself. You have made the earth your true home. And you can now help others to do the same by simply being who you are and have always been and by leading your life in a way that supports and honors the sacred balance of all things. But, remember, there is no finish line. As women we are labyrinths, continually winding our way to the center and back out again. Our lives are endless processes of becoming. May each season, each heartbreak, each birth, each death, each sunrise and sunset remind you to live fully, feel fully, and digest everything through your heart. It's not always easy, but it's the only way to truly come alive. When you forget, you can always start again. What's in the Way is the Way. The path is here. The Way is *in* you!

Epilogue

I remember riding on the train from Delhi to Agra to visit the Taj Mahal during my first trip to India. Although I had been living in Asia for nearly two years, I wasn't prepared for what I saw as I looked out the window that morning: shanty homes made out of sticks and bits of ragged cloth, propped up beside a river flowing with dirty plastic and brown sludge. In the homes and by the riverbanks, however, were what really surprised me: children laughing and playing, women smiling as they dipped their laundry into the soiled stream, and jewel-colored saris blowing like noble flags on clothing lines. How could it be that people who had so little could be so happy?

Years later I heard a story about the Red Cross visiting some of the natives in Patagonia. They met with an elder medicine woman from the community who explained that, for them, health was a state of respect, and, in order to have it, certain things — belonging to the plants, trees, and humans — must come together to serve as their medicine. These included water, true and balanced words, good food, not talking over other people, the forest, the animals, the fish, harmony, the village community, having conversations with one another, keeping their ancient ways of life, respecting both their culture and individual selves, the vigor that comes from all the above-mentioned things, the secure living on the land, the family, the festivals. She explained that when the outsiders came and made them believe that they were dependent on money and material things, their healthy state was destroyed. "You talk badly of others and take our land, and no land means nothing to eat, and nothing to eat means illness, and in the end you pull out of your pockets a little white pill and want to make us believe that if we eat that pill, this pill means health. Is that really what you think health is?"

Your path from now on is to continue to find ways to protect your sacred, inner medicine. This medicine consists of happiness in simplicity — regardless of material objects — and living authentically by telling the truth about what it means to live in harmonious relationship with yourself, your family, your community, and the magic of the natural world that is in dire need of our love and support. Like you, the earth wants to renew herself. She also wants us to trust, as she does, in the ever-changing seasons of our hearts and lives. She longs for us to return to wholeness by growing more comfortable with change and by remembering the bigger picture of our mysterious and vast interconnectedness.

Many seeds that you've planted have not yet blossomed. Remember that true change begins at the unseen levels first — like seeds burrowed way down in the dark, wet earth. Let all your efforts, dreams, and prayers keep incubating. Don't give up on them. Water them with your loving awareness, and trust that they will come into being in their own divine timing.

As I complete the final revisions for this book it's January, and I'm back in Chiang Mai — twelve years after having visited here for the first time. The

FINAL CONTEMPLATIONS

To help you navigate your transition with wisdom and self-knowing, here are some final contemplations for you:

1. I now rank my current priorities as follows: (Put a number next to each of the categories below. Feel free to tweak them to make them more relevant if needed.)
    ___ friends
    ___ finances
    ___ romance
    ___ health
    ___ spirituality
    ___ personal growth
    ___ career
    ___ family
    ___ community
2. The main things that now bring me joy and really make my soul sing include _____, _____, _____, and, most of all, _____.
3. The thing about myself that I most learned to love and accept this year was:
4. My biggest fear about moving forward right now is _____. Some ideas that I have about how to be supported in facing that fear are:
5. The five things that I now know about being the woman I am that I didn't realize before are:
6. The three main things that I will be sure to take with me from this journey into the future are _____, _____, and _____ because _____.

bougainvillea still blooms outside, the birds still sing as they did then. But now I'm a completely different person, having gone through so many deaths and re-births in the past decade. I know in every cell of my being that everything I've shared with you in this book is what has empowered me to let go and evolve. On this balmy winter morning it's from the grounded and open body and heart of a joyous and free woman that I say good-bye to you (for now). Yes, it's been a journey arriving at this season in my life, but all the effort has been worth it. I am, without a doubt, a *truly* happy woman.

You too have developed so much awareness this year — of yourself, of your relationship to nature and your own cycles, and of the world around you. So be-fore we part ways, I want to offer some final advice. First, stay awake for your life. Don't fall asleep to her beauty. Keep your newfound freshness, your child-like curiosity, with you always. Don't take anything for granted. Second, let your heart expand and contract as it will — just as your breath, the ocean, and the cosmos do. Don't ever let it shut down again. Vow to yourself to keep your heart open, to always choose love — first for yourself and then for others — even if it hurts. Always remember that this is the only way. Find the beauty in all things. Celebrate it. Play your part in bringing joy and respect back into our world.

And, last, stay connected. Keep praying. Keep listening to your inner guid-ance. Keep writing in your journal and reaching out to other women. Seek out mentors, coaches, teachers, role models, and women's circles to help you con-tinue to grow and evolve. There are lots of way that The Way of the Happy Woman community can be here for you — whether through joining one of our circles (virtual or live), coming on retreat, or taking a longer training pro-gram. Remember, you don't ever need to do anything alone. You are an in-tegral thread in the divine web of life. The more you recognize that web, the more it can be there to support you. Play your part in ending the era of isolation and reclaiming the power of the tribe. Know your place in that, and continue to show up for your family and your community.

And as we each stand as who we truly are in different places on this earth, I feel so much gratitude for who you are and the tremendous work that you've done on this journey. May you continue to reflect the things that your soul deeply values, and may your presence in this world help to heal and uplift oth-ers. Keep shining your light. Keep moving those mountains. And keep becom-ing more and more of the woman you came here to be.

May you be happy, and may the teachings shared in this book be of benefit to you and all beings.

Acknowledgments

This book was born out of love, not only my own but that of the countless people who have graced my life.

First, I thank the Divine Mother, who for me is always Mother Nature. We did this together, and you certainly took the lead. Thank you for showing me the way and for teaching me how to listen to your continual whispers in my ear.

I thank my parents, Sara Hatton Stover and Richard Robert Stover. I love you both so much. Mom, you've been with me through it *all*, and there are no words for that. Papa, thank you for still calling me Bear, for your big hugs, and for modeling discipline and perseverance. Thank you both for supporting my offbeat path.

Thank you to my three sisters, Shaw Stover Ruder, Christian Stover, and Anne Stover. You are all beautiful, unique, and amazing. We've been through so much together, and you are my best friends. Also thank you to my two beautiful nephews, Beckett and Elliot Ruder (and my new niece or nephew on the way), who remind me how to play and show me how big my capacity to love really is. Thank you also, Chris Ruder, for all that you bring to our family.

I give great thanks to my late grandparents, Sara Jane Avant Hatton (Mimi) and Frances Christian Hatton (Gaga). I miss you both so much, but your love and encouragement were so profuse that they're in me forever!

I also bow deeply to my teachers: ShantiMayi, Sofia Diaz, Richard Freeman, Sarah and Ty Powers; my first yoga teacher, Roberta; the Buddha, dharma, and the sangha; and Mother Maya. I extend much gratitude to the virtual dharma teachings of Jack Kornfield and Tara Brach, which I listened to on many mornings while writing this book. Thank you to those luminaries in women's yoga, spirituality, and health who have inspired me: Indra Devi, Gita Iyengar, Angela Farmer, Clarissa Pinkola Estés, Lama Tsultrim Allione, Bobby Clennell, Nischala Joy Devi, Vanda Scaravelli, Dr. Christiane Northrup, and

Gurmukh Kaur Khalsa. Thank you to the grandmother medicine, Alberto Martinez, and Harmony Sue Haynie — who continue to help me heal and expand my vision.

Thank you, Anand Mehrotra and Dr. Katyayani Poole, for your insightful Jyotisha readings over the years. I cannot even begin to tell you how much they have helped me to navigate my life and dharma. Also, thank you Diana Manilova and Marc Cofer for your intuitive guidance when I needed it most. Alexandra Shenpen, your humor and wisdom have helped me to find my own, and Maggie Staedler, your acupuncture, intuitive touch, and magical homeopathic potions helped heal my body and heart while I was writing this book.

A great web of friends and colleagues helped me in various ways through my book-writing journey. Deva Munay, your friendship saved me. Thank you for being my book midwife and for being the wild, wonderful medicine woman you are. D'vorah Swarzman, your friendship saved me too! Thank you for welcoming me to Ashland with open arms and for providing me with such a beautiful, creative space in which I could heal and write this book. Patrice Shakti Bacal, thank you for your kiva and for being my book doula in the final days, helping me to push this out when I didn't think I could. Also, thank you for your support, in various ways: Kari Nelson, Tracey Holderman, Maria Craven, Susanna Nicholson, Joung-ah Ghedini-Williams, Peach Friedman Dumars, Heidi Rose Robbins, Gail Larsen, Mary Taylor, Ren Resch, Elysabeth Williamson, Rebecca Andrist, Esther White, Mel Campbell, Lucas Rockwood, Joan Anderson, Rosemary Carstens, Beth Hayden, Sara Bercholz, Amy Olson Goin, Deborah Billig Scheck, Jennifer Lee, Amber Kinney, Deborah Fryer, Jeanie Manchester, Susan Manchester, Chameli Ardagh, Sabrina Chaw, Keith Martin-Smith, Dave Payne, Annie Platt, and Ellin Todd.

I'm also grateful to my Chiang Mai and Thailand community, especially Dr. Rungrat, Hillary Adrian Hitt, Rosemary Bolivar, Leslie Nguyen Temple, Silky Piehler, Pierre Whittman, and Lauren Brown.

Also, thank you to those who supported my writing during various stages of life, especially Dr. Ed Gomez, Dr. Rosalind Rosenberg, and Brian Larkin. Thank you, Susan Piver: your writing and meditation retreat at Shambhala Mountain Center helped to catapult me into this whole book-writing process with grace, depth, and ease.

Thank you to Barnard College for giving me such a unique and empowering all-women's education and to Ricki Booker of Ladies Who Launch for holding the space for me to manifest this vision. Thank you to my past teachers, Susan Warren (ballet) and Kali Franciska Von Koch (meditation). Thank you, Jan King, for being such an encouraging book coach, Francine Ward for your legal savvy, Georgia Hughes for being such a collaborative and wise editor, Molly O'Brien for your beautiful illustrations, Tracy Cunningham for a gorgeous cover, Kim Corbin for all your help with publicity, Kristen Cashman for your keen eye, Tona Pearce Myers for your careful typesetting, Mimi Kusch for your copyediting genius, and the entire New World Library team who helped bring this book into being. I send gratitude to Julia Cameron and her book *The Artist's Way*, which helped me to get unstuck creatively and bring this whole thing into being in the first place. Thank you to the trails of Mt. Sanitas and the vast skies of Boulder that held and inspired me day after day.

I also thank my guides, who continue to show me the way, especially Vajra Yogini, Machig Labdron, Saraswati, Mary Magdalene, and archangels Michael and Raphael. Thank you to the healing waters of Lake Michigan and the Ganga. Also, I thank my little girl muse, Pippi Longstocking, for reminding me to always march to the beat of my own drum and never leave my spunk behind.

Finally, I thank all the women who have shared their stories and opened their bodies and hearts with me over the years. It's been a complete honor and pleasure. I bow to each and every one of you.

INTRODUCTION

1. Elizabeth Gilbert, *Eat, Pray, Love: One Woman's Search for Everything across Italy, India and Indonesia* (New York: Viking, 2006), 260.

CHAPTER 1. KEEP IT SIMPLE

1. Louann Brizendine, *The Female Brain* (New York: Morgan Road Books, 2006), 14.
2. Thomas Crook, "The Natural Love Drug." Available at http://www.mindfood.com/at-natural-love-drug-happiness-family-friends.seo.
3. Gale Berkowitz, "UCLA Study on Friendship among Women." Available at http://www.anapsid.org/cnd/gender/tendfend.html.

CHAPTER 2. THE CYCLES THAT HEAL

1. Maya Tiwari, *Ayurveda: Secrets of Healing* (Twin Lakes, WI: Lotus Press, 1995), 86.

CHAPTER 3. A WOMAN'S INNER WORLD

1. Albert Einstein. Available at http://thinkexist.com/quotation/the_intuitive_mind_is_a_sacred_gift_and_the/15585.html.
2. Sarah Powers, *Insight Yoga* (Boston: Shambhala, 2008), 25.

CHAPTER 7. IN THE KITCHEN: CLEAN AND GREEN

1. Melanie Murray, "The 'Dirty Dozen' of Produce," *Environmental Working Group* (June 9, 2007). Available at http://ewg.org/node/21700.

CHAPTER 15. IN THE KITCHEN: ROOT WISDOM

1. Amanda D. Cueller and Michael E. Webber, "Wasted Food, Wasted Energy: The Embedded Energy in Food Waste in the United States," *Environmental Science & Technology* (July 21, 2010). Available at http://pubs.acs.org/stoken/presspac/presspac/abs/10.1021/es100310d.

2.   "A Mealtime Blessing from Thich Nhat Hanh." Available at http://pubs.acs.org/stoken/presspac/presspac/abs/10.1021/es100310d.

CHAPTER 16. ON THE YOGA MAT: GATHERING STRENGTH

1.   Jack Kornfield, *The Art of Forgiveness, Lovingkindness, and Peace* (New York: Bantam, 2008), 135.

CHAPTER 18. LISTENING

1.   Maya Tiwari, *Women's Power to Heal: Through Inner Medicine* (Candler, NC: Mother Om Media, 2007), 253–64.

CHAPTER 19. IN THE KITCHEN: STAYING WARM

1.   Nancy Kalish, "Super D," *O Magazine* 11 (November 2010): 134.

T

Sara Avant Stover is a motivational speaker, teacher, mentor, and founder and director of The Way of the Happy Woman®. The second oldest of four sisters and a Phi Beta Kappa and summa cum laude graduate of Columbia University's Barnard College, Sara has spent her life delving into the center of her feminine heart while inspiring and empowering others along the way. She took her first yoga class at age eighteen and sat her first Buddhist meditation retreat a few years later, and knew immediately that she would devote her life to helping others discover their own indestructible happiness within. After a health scare in her early twenties, Sara moved to Chiang Mai, Thailand, where she lived for nine years, embarked on an extensive healing and spiritual odyssey throughout Asia, and, as a multicertified yoga teacher, served as one of the Western pioneer yoga teachers in that part of the world. Since then she has studied with many spiritual masters and has taught three thousand students in more than a dozen different countries. She directed the first two-hundred-hour yoga teacher training in northern Thailand and the first ever women's yoga teacher training in the world. Her work has been featured in *The Huffington Post, Yoga Journal, Fit Yoga, Pilates Style*, and *Yogi Times*. A lover of autumn, good sleep, beautiful shoes, and dark chocolate, Sara continues to travel the world leading women's workshops, retreats, and teacher trainings. When she's not living out of her suitcase, she calls the mountains of Boulder, Colorado, home. Visit Sara online at www.saraavantstover.com; she would love to hear from you!

ABOUT THE WAY OF THE HAPPY WOMAN®:

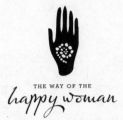

THE WAY OF THE
happy woman

The Way of the Happy Woman® helps modern women find unconditional happiness from the inside out through simplifying, slowing down, and reclaiming their cyclical natures.

This path offers something for women of all levels around the world: workshops, retreats, trainings, group and individual mentoring, and online products and programs. Sara is also available to speak to your group or organization about reclaiming women's health, wholeness, and happiness.

To find out more and to stay connected with The Way of the Happy Woman through our mailing list, you can visit us at:

www.SaraAvantStover.com
www.TheWayoftheHappyWoman.com
www.Facebook.com/WayofHappyWoman
www.Twitter.com/WayofHappyWoman